HORIZONS IN NEUROSCIENCE RESEARCH

VOLUME 35

HORIZONS IN NEUROSCIENCE RESEARCH

Additional books in this series can be found on Nova's website under the Series tab.

Additional e-books in this series can be found on Nova's website under the eBooks tab.

HORIZONS IN NEUROSCIENCE RESEARCH

VOLUME 35

ANDRES COSTA
AND
EUGENIO VILLALBA
EDITORS

nova biomedical
New York

Library of Congress Cataloging-in-Publication Data

ISBN: 978-1-53613-286-1
ISSN:2159-113X

Published by Nova Science Publishers, Inc. † New York

Contents

PREFACE

In this compilation, the authors explore novel strategies for enhancing efficacy of SAHA in combination with other anti-tumor drugs. Although SAHA is used against various types of cancer cells, it still does not show high efficacy as a monotherapy against solid tumors, therefore new strategies must be explored for induction of growth arrest, differentiation, and apoptosis in different preclinical models of glioblastoma. The authors go onto address motion-induced blindness, which occurs when a stationary foreground pattern is not or only partially perceived due to a moving background pattern although it is not obscured by the moving background pattern. Two studies are presented which illustrate the motion-induced blindness and spinning dancer paradigms. This book also examines childhood maltreatment, the most frequent form of trauma during early childhood. In people exposed to maltreatment in childhood, numerous neurobiological changes have been found, primarily in the neuroendocrine systems activated by stress, which include the function of the autonomous nervous system and the hypothalamic–pituitary–adrenal ax. Continuing, this book summarizes and discusses the findings of existing literature characterizing the normal biomechanics of the tibial nerve and comparing the normal biomechanics of this nerve against its biomechanics in the presence of pathology. This is done by synthesizing existing evidence on ultrasound applied in the study of different pathologies that can affect peripheral nerves, as well as the development of new procedures and technologies for a better nerve biomechanics characterization. A chapter is included which discusses the role of functional neuroimaging for research on ICDs and disinhibition in Parkinson's Disease. Significant neuropsychological and neuroanatomical data is analyzed, focusing on the concept of "motor impulsivity" in terms of "disinhibition of prepotent responses". Later, the authors present a study with the goal of making an accurate cell quantification of retinal ganglion cells by comparing two types of retrograde axonal transport in RGCs. The basics of neurobiology and neuropsychology, learning processes and forming of neural connections to the brain are presented. The current knowledge of vessel wall MRI in the assessment of intracranial aneurysms is also reviewed. This new technique offers the potential to assess both ruptured and unruptured aneurysms at the level of the wall and underlying pathology that has hitherto been impossible to do with standard luminal imaging techniques such as angiography. The concluding chapter summarizes the current knowledge on the timing, risk factors and management of aneurysmal rebleeding, as there remains significant controversy regarding the risk factors, pathophysiology and optimal treatment to prevent rebleeding.

Chapter 1 - Histone deacetylase (HDAC) enzymes cause epigenetic changes and thereby regulate gene expression in higher eukaryotic cells. Removal of the acetyl group (CH3CO-) from ε-N-acetyl lysine of the core histone proteins by HDAC can lead to tumor development and progression. This epigenetic modification should be explored and targeted for controlling growth of tumors. HDAC inhibitors are promising new therapeutic drugs for inhibiting growth of aggressive tumors by inducing cell cycle arrest, differentiation, and apoptosis in the tumor cells. Interestingly, HDAC inhibitors have shown cytotoxic effects against tumor cells, which are resistant to conventional chemotherapeutic agents. Suberoylanilide hydroxamic acid (SAHA), which is a potent pan-HDAC inhibitor, has been tested in different malignancies in vitro as well as in vivo. So far, SAHA has shown modest effects as a monotherapy for growth arrest and apoptosis in glioblastoma, which is the most prevalent and malignant brain tumor in humans. The mechanism of action of SAHA is due to its direct binding to zinc (Zn^{2+}) in the active site of HDAC leading to accumulation of acetylation, down regulation of anti-apoptotic Bcl-2 protein, and upregulation of pro-apoptotic Bax protein. Low dose of SAHA activates caspase-8 and p53 for inducing apoptosis. Some recent studies have shown a high ability of SAHA in promoting differentiation in glioblastoma cells. Also, SAHA slows down glioblastoma growth by modulation of autophagy. Although SAHA is used against various types of cancer cells, it still does not show high efficacy as a monotherapy against solid tumors. Therefore, novel strategies for enhancing efficacy of SAHA in combination with other anti-tumor drugs must be explored for induction of growth arrest, differentiation, and apoptosis in different preclinical models of glioblastoma.

Chapter 2 - Motion-induced blindness occurs when a stationary foreground pattern is not or only partially perceived due to a moving background pattern although it is not obscured by the moving background pattern. Periods of blindness alternate with periods of clear perception. Perception is oscillatory. Likewise, the so-called spinning dancer movie presenting a silhouetted rotating dancer figure induces oscillatory perception. Periods in which the dancer is perceived to rotate clockwise alternate with periods in which the dancer is perceived to rotate counter-clockwise although during both periods the movie plays the same frames. Two experiments are reported to illustrate the motion-induced blindness and spinning dancer paradigms. Subsequently, a neuronal network approach is presented to explain the oscillatory perceptual dynamics. The neuronal network approach is based on synergetics, a theory of pattern formation and self-organization. Accordingly, the theoretical framework explains perceptual oscillations in terms of a self-regulated alternation of brain activity patterns.

Chapter 3 - Childhood maltreatment is the most frequent form of trauma during early childhood, which may cause numerous difficulties, both in childhood and in adulthood. This chapter gives an overview of research so far into the effect of maltreatment in childhood on structural and functional changes to various parts of the nervous system. In people exposed to maltreatment in childhood numerous neurobiological changes have been found, primarily in the neuroendocrine systems activated by stress, which include the function of the autonomous nervous system, and the hypothalamic–pituitary–adrenal axis. The consequences of maltreatment in childhood are also evident in the prefrontal cortex region of the brain, as well as in various parts of the limbic system. Research also reports the negative effects of maltreatment on the development of the corpus callosum. The results of research so far indicate that when studying the effect of traumatic experience, such as maltreatment in childhood, the many factors involved must not be overlooked, such as the developmental period when the maltreatment occurred, the child's sex, and the severity and form of maltreatment to which the child was exposed. These factors separately, but also their interactive effects, may change the mechanism of the effects of maltreatment on neurobiological processes.

Chapter 4 - Nerves in general and the tibial nerve in particular are able to respond to movement and sustained postures while maintaining their normal function. They adapt to these stresses through a variety of mechanisms, such as gliding in relation to adjacent structures, increased strain and ability to tolerate compression. These mechanisms are named nerve biomechanics. Nevertheless, it is believed that nerve biomechanics is impaired in the presence of pathology and some health professionals, such as physiotherapists, make an attempt to restore it as a means to restore normal nerve function. However, for a comprehensive understanding of the normal tibial nerve biomechanics and how it is affected by pathology there is a need to i) characterize normal tibial nerve biomechanics, ii) changes in tibial nerve biomechanics in the presence of pathology and iii) whether these changes relate to changes in the tibial nerve function. Furthermore, nerve biomechanics is usually characterized through medical imaging studies, namely in ultrasound scoop. There is some variability associated with the performance of the ultrasound studies, which is very dependent on the equipment used, but also on the study protocol, on the equipment used, as well as on the experience and preferences of the observer, what makes it difficult to select the most appropriate strategies to characterize tibial nerve biomechanics using ultrasonography. Therefore, this chapter aims to i) characterize normal and pathological nerve biomechanics and how these can be used to inform non-invasive interventions directed at restoring normal nerve function using joint movement and ii) to critically analyze measurement procedures, image characterization and its reliability characteristics. This will be achieved by summarizing and discussing the findings of existing literature characterizing normal biomechanics of the tibial nerve and comparing the normal biomechanics of this nerve against its biomechanics in the presence of pathology and by synthetizing existing evidence on ultrasound applied in the study of different pathologies that can affect peripheral nerves, namely in their performance, as well as the development of new procedures and technologies for a better nerve biomechanics characterization. The authors will also discuss the clinical implications of their findings, in particular for the use of neural mobilization, a technique commonly used by physiotherapists to treat pathology of the peripheral nerves.

Chapter 5 - Impulse Control Disorders (ICDs) are behavioral disturbances in which a person fails to resist the drive to behave in ways that result in distress or impaired social and occupational functioning. The incidence of ICDs in Parkinson's disease (PD) is as high as 20%. Dopamine agonists can induce alterations in those frontostriatal networks that manage reward and mediate impulse monitoring and control. Indeed, tonic stimulation of dopamine receptors may damage inhibitory control mechanisms and reward processing, while promoting compulsive repetition of behavior. ICDs have, in fact, been associated with depressed mood, disinhibition, irritability, and appetite disturbance. Moreover, many PD patients have difficulties with mental processing speed, response-inhibition, and shifting between different conceptual sets, suggesting frontal-executive dysfunction. The neurocognitive approach considers two measurable executive functions from which ICDs can be detected: 1) response-inhibition, which neural substrate is located in the inferior portion of the prefrontal cortex; 2) integration of reward/punishment contingencies in individual choices, which neural substrate is located in the orbital-prefrontal cortex. Establishing such a relationship between disinhibition and executive functions could potentially be helpful for therapeutic research and for the efficient targeting of symptom relief in PD. For this reason, the authors present the preliminary results of an fMRI study with the aim of exploring response-inhibition performance and the neural correlates of inhibition that varied on self-reported trait impulsivity. This chapter will discuss the role of functional neuroimaging for research on ICDs and disinhibition in PD. Significant neuropsychological and neuroanatomical data will be highlighted and attention will be drawn to the concept of "motor impulsivity" in terms of "disinhibition of prepotent responses.

Chapter 6 - *Background and objectives:* The visual system is an approachable part of the central nervous system, which is suitable for investigating neuronal death, as well as to develop therapies toward its prevention. Mouse visual pathway has been used as a model to study degenerative neurological disorders, especially after technology has allowed the generation of genetically engineered animals. To make an accurately cell quantification of retinal ganglion cells (RGCs) is one of the main objectives in these works, due to its high variability among diverse strains of mice. The goal of this study was to compare two types of retrograde axonal transport in RGCs. *Material and methods:* After anaesthetizing the mouse, the midline of skin, on the top of head, was cut, and small holes were made in the skull following stereotactic localization of *superior colliculi.* Following withdrawal of a tiny portion of bone, part of the cerebral cortex was aspirated and the *superior colliculi* were exposed, placing a sponge soaked in the retrograde tracer Fluorogold on its surface. One week later, under anesthesia, after cutting the left superior rectus and left superior oblique eye muscles, the optic nerve was dorsally exposed and cut. Then, a piece of spongostan soaked in dextran tetramethyl rhodamine (DTMR) was applied on the optic nerve stump to label RGCs. At different post-labeling times, eyes were enucleated and the retinas fixed and mounted to study. Left retinas (injured) were analyzed with both labeling, FG and DTMR; while right retinas (uninjured) were only observed under FG labeling. *Results and discussion:* Different tracers stained RGCs in a different way. FG-labeled RGCs had a typical bright punctate and diffuse blue fluorescence, delineating their soma and the initial portion of their primary dendrites; while DTMR labeled cells had a red bright fluorescence. Counts of DTMR labeling cells were less numerous than FG labeling cells. Probably, it was due to a problem in axonal transport after injury. Also, some RGCs were labeled only with DTMR. It could be explained because there is a minority of RGCs that project to other nuclei different to *superior colliculi.* After optic nerve injury, a progressive decrease in RGCs number and an increase in microglial cells number were observed. When labeled RGCs are phagocytosed by microglial cells, tracer was incorporated into the microglial cell and become fluorescent. *Conclusion:* Different tracers and different places to apply along the visual pathways must be considered depending on the specific characteristics required by the project being carried out.

Chapter 7 - The aim of the article is to present the basics of neurobiology and neuropsychology, learning processes and forming of neural connections in the brain. The author of the article utilizes knowledge of neurobiology and neuropsychology which are currently part of neuroscience. She describes sensitive periods, also referred to as critical, as periods during which particular neural networks grow more rapidly and numerous synaptic connections are formed. What occurs then is synaptogenesis, which is the base of development of links among cells making the brain more flexible and capable of learning faster. Then she describes the process of learning on the neurophysiological level. The author highlights certain critical periods in the development of children. They include touch sensitivity, recognizing faces, sound categorization leading to language learning, ability to count and motion sensitivity. Further in the article, the author refers to the concept of Maria Montessori, which, in certain aspects, is consistent with the occurrence of sensitive periods. Celestyna Grzywniak emphasizes the significance of early teaching of children and enriching their environment by introducing appropriate activities. She draws attention to stimulation of neural links through environment, which should be specially enriched by applying appropriate stimuli. The article emphasizes the need to repeatedly apply effective stimuli in order to enhance the flow of nerve impulses and clear up nerve pathways.

Chapter 8 - Advanced imaging techniques have allowed intracranial aneurysms to be examined under ever-closer scrutiny. Whilst some of these imaging techniques are still at the research stage others have entered clinical practice. One technique in particular holds much promise and could enter routine use in hospital practice with relative ease. This new technique, that allows assessment of the vessel wall and aneurysm wall offers the potential to assess both ruptured and unruptured aneurysms at the level of the wall and underlying pathology that has hitherto been impossible to do with standard luminal imaging techniques such as angiography. In this review the authors discuss the current knowledge of vessel wall MRI in the assessment of intracranial aneurysms. Contrast enhanced vessel wall MRI is a state-of –the-art technique that aims to assess the vessel wall and provide real time in vivo pathological level imaging. To successfully image the intracranial vessel walls one needs to suppress the intra-arterial signal from the blood – the so-called black blood technique. This is essential in order to attain sufficient image contrast to enable accurate assessment and interpretation of the vessel wall. However, this can be a difficult task given that the angulation of the blood vessels is extremely variable which means sufficient suppression of the blood signal can be challenging. A variety of different methods have been used to obtain black blood imaging and these include the use of motion sensitizing pre-pulses and double inversion recovery techniques. It is also important to suppress the CSF signal surrounding the vessels in order to allow a complete assessment of the arterial wall. However, a problem with CSF signal suppression is the resultant decrease in Signal-to-noise ratio (SNR) derived from the vessel wall itself. The combination of multiple suppression sequences and high resolution imaging can also mean prohibitively long scan times and increasing motion artefacts that cause image degradation. The small size of the intracranial vessels and the need for high spatial resolution with high SNR and acceptable scan times necessitates a reduced scan volume. This has in turn resulted in a focus on the circle of Willis and proximal intracranial vessels. Some investigators have opted for a lower spatial resolution to detect enhancement of the vessels secondary to the increase in contrast to noise ratio caused by contrast uptake. This approach may be useful to assess the generalized burden and anatomical distribution of a disease process. As mentioned earlier high SNR is essential for adequate assessment of the vessel wall. The introduction of 3Tesla machines into routine practice has meant improved SNR is now available and this can be used to either shorten scan times or improve spatial resolution. The availability of 7Tesla MR machines, although generally restricted to research institutions at the current time, will hopefully mean further similar improvements in spatial resolution and scan times can be made.

Chapter 9 - Aneurysmal rebleeding after initial subarachnoid hemorrhage is associated with very high morbidity and mortality. While some studies suggest rebleeding occurs in approximately 4% of patients within the first 24 hours after initial subarachnoid hemorrhage, these studies may have underestimated the incidence of ultra-early rebleeding. Furthermore, there remains significant controversy regarding the risk factors, pathophysiology and optimal treatment to prevent rebleeding. In this chapter the authors summarize the current knowledge on the timing, risk factors and management of aneurysmal rebleeding.

In: Horizons in Neuroscience Research
Editors: A. Costa and E. Villalba
ISBN: 978-1-53613-286-1

Chapter 1

ANTI-TUMOR EFFECTS OF HDAC INHIBITORS: NOVEL STRATEGIES FOR ENHANCING ANTI-TUMOR EFFICACY OF THE HDAC INHIBITOR SAHA FOR CONTROLLING GROWTH OF GLIOBLASTOMA

Firas Khathayer and Swapan K. Ray*
Department of Pathology, Microbiology, and Immunology,
University of South Carolina School of Medicine, Columbia, SC, US

ABSTRACT

Histone deacetylase (HDAC) enzymes cause epigenetic changes and thereby regulate gene expression in higher eukaryotic cells. Removal of

* Corresponding author: Swapan K. Ray, PhD, Professor, Department of Pathology, Microbiology, and Immunology, University of South Carolina School of Medicine, Building 2, Room C11, 6439 Garners Ferry Road, Columbia, SC 29209, US. Phone: 803-216-3420; Fax: 803-216-3428; E-mail: swapan.ray@uscmed.sc.edu.

the acetyl group (CH3CO-) from ε-N-acetyl lysine of the core histone proteins by HDAC can lead to tumor development and progression. This epigenetic modification should be explored and targeted for controlling growth of tumors. HDAC inhibitors are promising new therapeutic drugs for inhibiting growth of aggressive tumors by inducing cell cycle arrest, differentiation, and apoptosis in the tumor cells. Interestingly, HDAC inhibitors have shown cytotoxic effects against tumor cells, which are resistant to conventional chemotherapeutic agents. Suberoylanilide hydroxamic acid (SAHA), which is a potent pan-HDAC inhibitor, has been tested in different malignancies in vitro as well as in vivo. So far, SAHA has shown modest effects as a monotherapy for growth arrest and apoptosis in glioblastoma, which is the most prevalent and malignant brain tumor in humans. The mechanism of action of SAHA is due to its direct binding to zinc (Zn^{2+}) in the active site of HDAC leading to accumulation of acetylation, down regulation of anti-apoptotic Bcl-2 protein, and upregulation of pro-apoptotic Bax protein. Low dose of SAHA activates caspase-8 and p53 for inducing apoptosis. Some recent studies have shown a high ability of SAHA in promoting differentiation in glioblastoma cells. Also, SAHA slows down glioblastoma growth by modulation of autophagy. Although SAHA is used against various types of cancer cells, it still does not show high efficacy as a monotherapy against solid tumors. Therefore, novel strategies for enhancing efficacy of SAHA in combination with other anti-tumor drugs must be explored for induction of growth arrest, differentiation, and apoptosis in different preclinical models of glioblastoma.

INTRODUCTION

Brain tumor is a mass of abnormal glial cells, which grow uncontrollably and spread to the nearby brain tissue (Appin and Brat, 2015). The most common brain tumors are malignant gliomas (masses of abnormal astrocytes or/and oligodendrocytes) with a world-wide incidence of about 5 per 100,000 individuals/year (Bondy et al., 2008; Ferlay et al., 2013). Since malignant gliomas originate from abnormal glia (astrocytes, oligodendrocytes, or both), which are star-shaped cells with extended processes throughout the surrounding brain region, it is practically impossible to surgically remove the gliomas with their entire cellular network. A few remaining tumor cells, which infiltrate into the nearby brain region, can cause recurrence of the tumor. There are broadly two types of malignant brain tumors: primary brain tumors and secondary brain tumors. Primary brain tumors have more than 120 types and about 80% of all primary brain tumors are glioblastoma multiforme or simply called glioblastoma (Macenka and Olivi, 2011). Only 3-5% of glioblastoma patients survive longer than 3 years and nearly 100% of all tumors recur (Krex et al., 2007). It has been predicted that about 26,000 patients will be diagnosed with primary brain tumors and more than 53,000 patients will be diagnosed with non-malignant brain tumors in the United States (US) in 2017 (Ostrom et al., 2015). About 55% of malignant brain tumors occur in males, while 45% in females. Glioblastoma is the most common malignant brain tumor in older adults, less common in children, and more prevalent in white people than in black people (Ostrom et al., 2016). Glioblastoma is a grade IV malignant brain tumor that arises from astroglial cells after several genetic mutations or alterations in some tumor suppressor genes (e.g., *p53, PTEN, p16, TP53*) and also some oncogenes (e.g., *Akt*, *EGFR, PARK2*). Glioblastoma is one of the most aggressive of all malignancies in humans. It is practically an incurable brain tumor. It grows very rapidly due to its resistance to radiotherapy and chemotherapy, making its treatment almost always unsuccessful (Lathia et al., 2015). After surgical resection of glioblastoma, especially the glioblastoma stem cells (GSC) remaining in the nearby brain tissue are highly resistant to radiotherapy, chemotherapy, and immune recognition and they can easily and rapidly regrow the tumor (Bischof et al., 2017).

The recent studies have demonstrated that development of glioblastoma is associated with a decrease in acetyl group in core histone proteins and non-histone proteins as well (Lucio-Eterovic et al., 2008). Histone deacetylase (HDAC) is the enzyme that is responsible for regulation of histone acetylation by removing acetyl groups (CH_3CO-) from the core histone proteins (Di Marcotullio et al., 2011), leading to chromatin condensation and transcriptional repression of the tumor suppressor genes (Kumagai et al., 2007). There are 18 mammalian HDAC enzymes and they are divided into four classes (I, II, III, and IV) (Table 1). The expression of the HDAC class I (1, 2, 3, 8), II (5, 6, 7, 9, and 10), and IV has been documented in glioblastoma (Lucio-Eterovic et al., 2008).

Surgery alone cannot cure glioblastoma because it does not remove all glioblastoma cells from the brain. Moreover, surgery is not an option if the tumor is deep within brain or in the brain stem. Genetic alterations and epigenetic modifications might contribute to aberrations in the apoptotic pathways in glioblastoma cells and thus confer resistance to radiotherapy and conventional chemotherapy. Besides, radiotherapy and conventional chemotherapy become meaningless due to side effects and limited results (Bukowska et al., 2015). So, there is an urgent need to develop novel therapeutic strategies that can inhibit activity of HDAC enzymes (Zhao et al., 2005) for accumulation of acetylation in histone proteins for expression of tumor suppressors (Shabason et al., 2011) in glioblastoma.

High anti-tumor effects of HDAC inhibitors promote cell death by G2 checkpoint abrogation leading to mitotic catastrophe in glioblastoma cells and other cancer cells, which are resistant to conventional drugs (Cornago et al., 2014). HDAC inhibitors either alone or synergistically with other inhibitors emerge as one of the newest promising classes of an anti-tumor drugs for treatment of glioblastoma (Kim and Bae, 2011). These inhibitors are able not only to target histone proteins in cancer cells but also they can show several biological effects such as cell cycle arrest, promotion of differentiation, and inhibition of angiogenesis in many cancer cells by preventing the removal of the acetyl groups from core histone proteins and also non-histone proteins such as transcription factors (e.g., p53, E2F1, STAT) and cytoplasmic proteins (e.g., α-tubulin, HSP90, and Ku70), consequently causing accumulation of acetyl groups or hyper acetylation (Glozak et al., 2005; Marks, 2007). Suberoylanilide hydroxamic acid (SAHA), which is an important pan-HDAC inhibitor, has been effective in causing cell death in glioblastoma and it has little negative effects on normal cells (Eyüpoglu et al., 2005). SAHA suppresses activities of the class I and class II HDAC via attachment of hydroxamic end of SAHA to Zn^{2+} in tubular pocket at active site of the target HDAC and carbon ring group of SAHA projects out of the pocket on surface of HDAC (Marks et al., 2001; Rickon, 2006), blocking the enzyme and causing increases in the acetylated histone and non-histone proteins such as p53 that bind DNA for transcription of tumor suppressors (Marks, 2007). SAHA has been approved by the US Food and Drug Administration (FDA) in October 2006 for treatment of cutaneous T cell lymphoma (Mann et al., 2007).

Table 1. Classification and action of human HDAC enzymes in brain according to their homology with yeast HDAC enzymes

	HDAC enzymes			
	Class I	Class II	Class III	Class IV
HDAC member(s)	HADC1, -2, -3, and -8	HADC4, -5, -7, and -9 (Class IIA); HDAC6 and -10 (Class IIB)	Sirt1-7	11
Cellular location	Nucleus/ cytoplasm	Nucleus/ cytoplasm	Nucleus	Nucleus
Protein complex	Sin3, CoREST, NuRD	Foxp3	-	HADC6
Cellular function	Repression of gene expression and differentiation	Induction of cell growth and self-renewal	Initiation, progression of tumor, and suppression of apoptosis	Cell proliferation
Localization in brain cells	Neuronal and glial cells	Glioblastoma and neural stem cells	Glioblastoma cells	Oligodendro cytes and some neurons
Target substrate	p21, Histones	p53, Rb, Histones, α-Tubulin, HSP90	Rb, Histones	Histones
Ion or molecule for activity	Zn^{2+}	Zn^{2+}	NAD^{+}	NAD^{+}
Binding with transcription factor	CREB	n-Myc, c-Myc, Myb, MEF2, TLX	-	-
Associated with transcriptional repressor	NCoR	NCoR, BCoR CtBP, SMRT	-	-
Catalytic site	1	1	-	2

However, SAHA is a double-edged sword in the context of autophagy in glioblastoma. SAHA alone causes tumor growth slowdown and triggers autophagy in GSC by down regulation of the autophagy inhibitory Akt/mTOR signaling, upregulation of the autophagy promoting Beclin-1 and LC3 II levels, and decrease in sequestosome 1 (SQSTM1, also known as p62) level (Chiao et al., 2013). Autophagy acts as a pro-survival mechanism by elimination of the damaged mitochondria and organelles from the tumor cells in aggressive tumors. Although SAHA alone activates autophagy via inhibiting mTOR and upregulating LC3 II expression in human glioblastoma T98G cells, inhibition of autophagy by RNAi results in an increase in SAHA-induced apoptosis in T98G cells, suggesting that combination of autophagy inhibition and SAHA treatment acts as a pro-apoptotic device in human glioblastoma (Gammoh et al., 2012).

One of the important ways to treat glioblastoma is the induction of differentiation in the tumor cells. SAHA can induce differentiation in the tumor cells so as to promote characteristics of the normal cells by increasing the level of p21Waf1/Cip1 for cell cycle arrest at G1 phase (Jones et al., 2009). SAHA has significant anti-glioblastoma effects as it induces cell cycle arrest and apoptosis via increased expression of anti-proliferative factors (e.g., p21Waf1/Cip1, p27Kip1, DR5, TNF-α) and the pro-apoptotic Bax protein, while it reduces expression of many cell cycle promoting proteins (e.g., CDK2, CDK4, Cyclin D1, Cyclin D2) and also the anti-apoptotic Bcl-2 protein (Yin et al., 2007). As a monotherapy, SAHA has only moderate anti-tumor activity in glioblastoma patients and additional testing of SAHA in combination regimens is warranted (Galanis et al., 2009). SAHA in combination with another anti-tumor agent should have more therapeutic effects against glioblastoma than when it is used as a monotherapy. Results reported from many studies in our laboratory demonstrated that a combination therapy was better than a monotherapy for controlling growth of human glioblastoma in vitro (Janardhanan et al., 2008; George et al., 2010; Chakrabarti et al., 2016) and also in vivo (George et al., 2009; George et al., 2010; Chakrabarti et al., 2013). Recent studies also suggest that the synergism of SAHA and another anti-tumor agent may facilitate its effectiveness in inhibiting growth of glioblastoma.

Combination of SAHA with another anti-tumor drug such as Temozolomide or Erlotinib can cause increase in killing of glioblastoma cells due to induction of apoptosis when compared with individual treatments, suggesting that in a combination setting, SAHA has a better ability to kill glioblastoma cells than a standard therapy (Banelli et al., 2015; Rasmusseen et al., 2016).

HDAC Enzymes and Their Roles in Formation and Progression of Glioblastoma

Cells need to coil and uncoil DNA around core histone proteins for regulation of gene expression. The regulation of gene expression occurs by a balance between histone acetylation and deacetylation levels. As an important epigenetic mechanism, histone modification plays a vital role in regulating gene expression and aberration in this process is responsible for occurrence of many diseases including cancers (Chen et al., 2015). Increased level of histone acetylation (hyper acetylation) induced by histone acetyltransferases (HAT) leads to activation of transcription of the gene due to induction of weakness in ionic relation between the negatively charged DNA backbone and the positively charged histone protein tails (Wade, 2001), while decreased level of histone acetylation (hypo acetylation) produced by HDAC activity is associated with silencing of gene expression (Mottamal et al., 2015). HAT can act to suppress or stimulate tumor growth. Acetylation of histones may make the DNA less condensed and thereby more transcription of the tumor suppressor genes.

HDAC enzymes are involved in epigenetic mechanisms for directly and indirectly controlling cellular processes including growth, inflammation, differentiation, and apoptosis (Lagger et al., 2002). HDAC reduces histone acetylation in core histone proteins by removing acetyl groups from ε-N-acetyl lysine from histone tails (Munster et al., 2011). Activity of HDAC thereby allows histones to wrap the DNA more tightly and prevent gene transcription (Struhl, 1998; Gallinari et al., 2007). Many studies have shown that HDAC plays a critical role in formation of cancers since this enzyme regulates expression and activity of several proteins associated with development and growth of cancers due to the condensed chromatin causing inhibition of transcription of the tumor suppressor genes. In addition, HDAC not only affects acetylation in chromatin histone proteins but also in non-histone proteins. HDAC regulates cell growth, differentiation, and apoptosis via repression of transcription factors, hormone receptors, chaperons, signal transducers, and other non-histone proteins (e.g., E2F, STAT3, p53, NF-κB, HSP90, α-tubulin, c-Myc, Rb) in the cells (Lin et al., 2006; Ropero and Esteller, 2007). For example, HDAC binds to the tumor suppressor protein p53 and removes acetyl group from its lysine residues, and this deacetylation inhibits p53 activation causing increase in cell proliferation (Juan et al., 2000). HDAC is also associated with regulation of Rb protein and represses gene transcription (Frolov and Dyson, 2004). Moreover, HDAC inhibits expression of p21 (also known as p21Waf1/Cip1), which is a key mediator of the p53-dependent cell cycle arrest, in different cell types and increase in HDAC activity is associated with decrease in expression of p21 in many cancers (Gui et al., 2004).

In mammalian cells, there are 18 different HDAC enzymes that are divided into four classes (I - IV) depending on their homology with auxiliary domains of the yeast HDAC enzymes (Li and Seto, 2016). The class I (which includes HDAC1, -2, -3 and -8), class IIA (which includes HDAC4, -5, -7 and -9), class IIB (which includes HDAC6 and -10), and class IV (which includes only HDAC11 that has features of both class I and II) enzymes require Zn^{2+} as co-factor in their active site for their deacetylation activity, while class III (which includes seven members known as the Sirtuins, namely Sirt1-7) enzymes need nicotinamide adenine dinucleotide (NAD^+, instead of Zn^{2+}) as co-factor for their enzymatic activity (Table 1) (Rikiishi, 2011; Chen et al., 2015). Among the class I enzymes, HDAC1, -2, and -3 are commonly found in cell nucleus in various human tissues, while HDAC8 is found in both nucleus and cytoplasm in glioblastoma and neuroblastoma (Liby et al., 2006; Retting et al., 2015). These enzymes are very important in regulating cell proliferation and survival (Park et al., 2008; Jung et al., 2012). HDAC1 and -2 are very similar enzymes in structure and function and they suppress apoptosis in tumor cells (Huang et al., 2005) and also they have negative effects on synaptic plasticity and formation of memory (Guan et al., 2009). Both enzymes are associated with other protein complexes such as Sin3 complex (a major mechanism to repress transcription in eukaryotic cells), NuRD (nucleosome remodeling deacetylase) complex, and the REST (repressor element-1 silencing transcription factor) corepressor (CoREST) to repress gene expression in neuronal cells and glial cells (MacDonald and Roskams, 2008). The nuclear receptor corepressors (NCoRs) are transcriptional repressors and found to be highly expressed and associated with HDAC1, -2, and -3 in glioblastoma cells (Campos, 2011). HDAC3 is mostly identical to HDAC8 in structure and function and it is different from other two class I (HDAC1 and -2) enzymes in transcriptional repression of p21Waf1/Cip1 (De Ruijter et al., 2003; Wilson et al., 2006). But it has been noticed that HADC3 forms complex with the corepressors NCoR and SMRT (silencing mediator for retinoid and thyroid receptors) that are different from other HDAC complexes for repression of expression of pro-apoptotic gene (Karagianni and Wong, 2007), while overexpression of HDAC8 significantly correlates with progression of neuroblastoma due to suppression of the cellular transcription factor CREB (cAMP response element-binding) mediated cell differentiation (Retting et al., 2015).

Class IIA (HDAC4, -5, -7, and -9) enzymes (Table 1) are expressed in specific human tissues (Weichert, 2009) and they can move between nucleus and cytoplasm (Marks, 2010). These enzymes link indirectly to DNA (Wang, 1999). A study has shown that overexpression of class II HDAC enzymes contribute to glioblastoma development and they are responsible for removing acetyl groups from histone H3 (Lucio-Eterovic et al., 2008). Also, it has been shown that class II HDAC enzymes are involved in increased expression of many oncoproteins (n-Myc, c-Myc, PDGFR, a-Myb, K-Ras, CDK4, EGFR, and MDM2) in glioblastoma, as these are found to be overexpressed in 40% of glioblastomas (Goussia, et al., 2000). HDAC4, -5, and -7 enzymes are present in same subgroup and have the ability to interact with transcriptional corepressors such as SMRT, NCoR, BCoR (BCL-6 interacting corepressor), CtBP (C-terminal-binding protein 1), and MEF2 (myocyte enhancer factor 2) to suppress gene expression and block muscle cell differentiation (Bertos et al., 2001), while they are found at low levels in glioblastoma (Lucio-Eterovic et al., 2008). HDAC5 contributes to neural stem cell proliferation by interaction with MEF2 and the transcription factor tailless (TLX, also known as the nuclear receptor NR2E1) to induce neural stem cell proliferation and self-renewal (Sun et al., 2007). HDAC9 belongs to a separate group although it is related to HDAC4, -5, and -7 enzymes and it appears to be in low level in glioblastoma but its expression increases in low-grade astrocytomas and normal brain cells (Lucio-Eterovic et al., 2008). It is involved in inhibition of differentiation of cortical cells in brain (Sugo et al., 2010). Class IIB (HDAC6 and -10) enzymes are responsible for deacetylation of α-tubulin and cortactin, which regulate microtubule and actin associated cell motility; HDAC6 is mostly a cytoplasmic enzyme that is involved in cell proliferation, promoting EGFR activity for glioblastoma development, and overexpression of HDAC6 confers resistance to Temozolomide in glioblastoma (Wang et al., 2016).

Class III enzymes are known as Sirtuins (Sirt) and there are seven types (Sirt1-7) in humans (Table 1), as mentioned above. These enzymes are highly regulated in brain tumor cells and may contribute to initiation and progression of the tumor and also apoptosis resistance (Liu et al., 2009). The results show that Sirt1, which is either upregulated or down regulated in glioblastoma, is a double-edged sword because it may act as tumor suppressor or as oncoprotein and it is found that Sirt1 may promote tumor by inducing PI3K/Akt signaling pathway or inhibit proliferation of glioblastoma cells via retardation of mitotic entry of the tumor cells and it may induce apoptosis by p53 and Rb (Qu et al., 2012). Sirt2 has been found to be overexpressed in human GSC and its activity effectively contributes to proliferation of human GSC and rat glioblastoma C6 cells by inhibition of caspase-3-dependent apoptotic pathway (He et al., 2012; Imaoka et al., 2012). Paradoxically, an opposing study demonstrated that overexpression of Sirt2 inhibited proliferation of human glioblastoma cells due to decrease in anti-apoptotic Bcl-2 level and increases in pro-apoptotic Bax and active caspase-3 levels (Li et al., 2013).

Class IV includes only HDAC11 enzyme that is similar to class I and class II enzymes in sequence and it is expressed more in oligodendrocytes and some neurons and increased during 1 day to 4 weeks (Liu et al., 2008). HDAC11, which is located in nucleus and cytoplasm, plays a key role in controlling expression and repression of genes in many types of cancer cells (Deubzer et al., 2013). An investigation has shown that class II and IV HDAC enzymes play important roles in regulation of histone modification in the brain and development of low-grade and high-grade astrocytomas while class I HDAC enzymes have hardly any effect on the tumor development (Lucio-Eterovic et al., 2008). In contrast, another study found that class I HADC1 enzyme could play a significant role in promotion of brain tumor (Rasmussen et al., 2016). The understanding of the functions of HDAC enzymes in glioblastoma may facilitate the finding ways to design and produce the anti-tumor drugs for inhibition of specific HDAC enzymes for successful treatment of glioblastoma.

Exploration of Different Groups of HDAC Inhibitors for Treatment of Glioblastoma

All classes of HDAC enzymes have many targets in histone and non-histone proteins leading to alterations in gene expression and thereby they can play roles in tumor development (Marks, 2007). HDAC inhibitors are natural and chemical compounds that have the ability to inhibit the activity of class I, II, and IV HDAC enzymes (Gregoretti et al., 2004; Drummond et al., 2005). They are the new anti-cancer drugs that bind to Zn^{2+} in active site of HDAC and inhibit its enzymatic activity leading to accumulation of acetylation in histone and non-histone proteins; consequently, they play active roles in cell growth inhibition by inducing transcription of the cell cycle arresting proteins such as p16, p21, and p27 (Nishida et al., 2004) and by promoting differentiation and also apoptosis with increases in expression of pro-apoptotic proteins such as Bax, Bid, and Bad in many types of cancer cells in vitro and in vivo (Zhang et al., 2004; Carew et al.,

2008). HDAC inhibition is known to significantly contribute to reductions in proliferation of cancer cells that resist the chemotherapeutic drugs by down regulating levels of G2 checkpoint kinases Wee1 and Chk1 (Cornago et al., 2014). HDAC inhibitors also down regulate vascular endothelial growth factor receptor (VEGFR) causing inhibition of growth of new blood vessels, which otherwise provide nutrient and oxygen for growth of tumor cells (Deroanne et al., 2002), while they increase generation of intracellular reactive oxygen species (ROS) to facilitate tumor cell death. They increase acetylation of HSP90 that leads to degradation of proteins that cause cancer (Rosato et al., 2003; Kim and Bae, 2011).

All HDAC inhibitors are currently categorized into at least four groups (Figure 1): hydroxamates, short chain fatty acids (SCFA), cyclic peptides, and benzamides (Marks and Breslow, 2007). Two pan-HDAC inhibitors are Trichostatin A (TSA) and SAHA (also called Vorinostat or Zolinza), which are hydroxamates and they have already been approval by the US FDA for using as drugs for treatment of various cancers (Duvic and Vu, 2007). Some HDAC inhibitors can inhibit specific type of HDAC; for example, TSA has strong inhibitory effect on all class I HADC enzymes, but MS-275 (a synthetic benzamide) is considered to be better in inhibiting HDAC1 than HDAC2 and -3 while it has shown no inhibitory effect on HDAC8 (Hu et al., 2003).

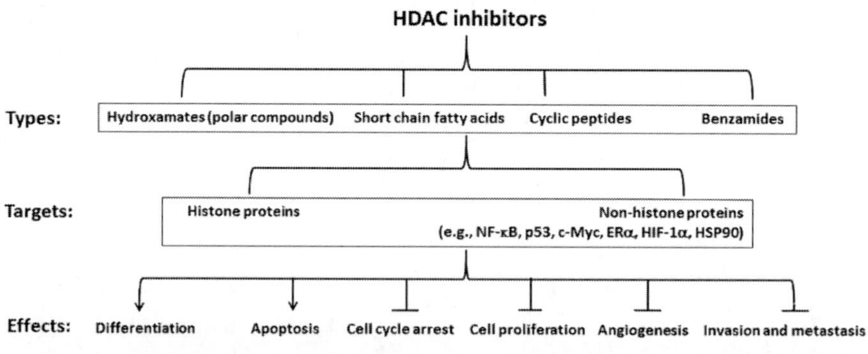

Figure 1. Main types of HDAC inhibitors that alter chromatin activities and several non-histone proteins leading to expression of genes for a wide spectrum of biological effects such as alterations in cell cycle, differentiation, apoptosis, and angiogenesis.

Hydroxamates are the well-studied first group of HDAC inhibitors. Hydroxamate-based hybrid polar compounds (HPCs) are novel molecules that can be used at micromolar or lower concentrations against cancers for promoting differentiation and apoptosis in vitro and in vivo, and these HDAC inhibitors have tubular structure that can bind to Zn^{2+} in the tubular pocket of active site of HDAC and thereby they can release carbon ring group to the outside pocket on the surface of the protein (Finnin et al., 1999). Generally, HPCs inhibit the activities of class I, II, and IV HADC enzymes (Abbas and Gupta, 2008) to repress growth of glioblastoma by accumulating acetylated histone. It has been observed that levels of acetylation in the core histones H2A, H2B, H3 and H4 are increased when the cancer cells are treated with HPCs (Bezecny, 2014). Histones H1 and H5 are linker histones. SAHA can be used at high dose as an effective chemotherapy for treatment of human glioblastoma in vitro and in vivo, while it at low dose has shown no major efficacy in inhibiting the growth of human glioblastoma (Yin et al., 2007). The results show that administration of SAHA (10 mg/kg) acts to accumulate the acetylated histones H3 and H4 resulting in upregulation of the cell cycle arresting proteins p21 and p27 and down regulation of cell cycling proteins (e.g., CDK2, CDK4, Cyclin D1, Cyclin D2) in glioblastoma xenografts. Increasing the dose of SAHA administration led to increase in suppression in tumor growth (Coffey et al., 2001; Yin et al., 2007). TSA, which is also one of the HPCs, has robust effects in glioblastoma. TSA plays critical role in inducing differentiation by increasing expression of glial fibrillary acidic protein (GFAP), which is an acclaimed astrocytic differentiation marker, and in inducing apoptosis by activating caspase-3 in different human glioblastoma cell lines GBM29, U343MG, and U343MG (Svechnikova et al., 2008). Also, TSA triggers innate immune responses against tumor cells by inducing expression of the natural killer group-2 member-D (NKG2D) ligands major histocompatibility complex class I-related chain (MIC)-A and UL16 binding protein (ULBP)-2 at mRNA and protein levels, making them susceptible to lysis by NK cells (Höring et al., 2013).

SCFA molecules are the next group of HDAC inhibitors, the structure of which has a relationship with inhibitory activity. Inhibitors having non-branching SCFA are better inhibitors than inhibitors that have a branch SCFA (Gilbert, 2006). For example, n-butyric acid that is one of the non-branching SCFA molecules has greater inhibitory activity than 2,2-dimethylbutyric acid having a branch SCFA (Boosalis et al., 2001). Butyric acid is primary fuel supplement of colon cells for controlling pH in the colon to inhibit growth of bacterial pathogens and repress inflammation in the colon (Adom and Nie, 2013). Butyric acid also has ability of arresting cell growth, restarting DNA synthesis, and inhibiting growth of colon cancer cells (Andriamihaja et al., 2009); it also plays critical role in induction of apoptosis and inhibition of proliferation of glioblastoma cells and it significantly attributes to caspase-8 activity mediated apoptosis (Komata et al., 2005). Valproic acid (VPA), which is one of the SCFA derivatives and produced by *Valeriana officinalis,* is widely used in the treatment of glioblastoma and VPA has been shown to have high capability of inducing differentiation and inhibiting cell growth by suppressing DNA repair, increasing cell cycle arrest at G2/M phase, and increasing ROS and expression of pro-apoptotic family proteins (Berendsen et al., 2012; Tseng et al., 2017). VPA reduces the activity and expression levels of matrix metalloproteinases (MMP2 and MMP9) and it is involved in the breakdown of extracellular matrix (ECM) proteins and blocking metastasis of glioblastoma (Papi et al., 2010). The studies show that its fatty acid chain causes the inhibitory activity in glioblastoma cells via two mechanisms: first, stimulation of the tumor suppressor p21 that induces cell cycle arrest at G1; second, fatty acid chain increases acetylation at chromatin by inhibiting HDAC enzyme so as to allow promotion of transcription of the tumor suppressor genes and consequently inhibition of carcinogenesis (Entin-Meer et al., 2005).

Cyclic peptides are another group of HDAC inhibitors and they have a variety of biological effects such as immunosuppression activity, anti-bacterial activity, and anti-tumor activity (Loffet, 2002). They are known to have the most complexity in structure than any other group of HDAC inhibitors (Miller et al., 2003). Cyclic peptides are prodrugs and have disulfide bond that is intracellularly reduced to thiol moiety to bind to Zn^{2+} in the active site pocket of class I HDAC enzymes (Yoshida et al., 2003).

They are divided into two subfamilies. The first subfamily includes cyclic tetrapeptides such as Apicidin, Trapoxin, Azumamide, and HC-toxin. The second subfamily includes bicyclic depsipeptide HDAC inhibitors (Townsend et al., 2007). The hydrophobic cyclic tetrapeptides contain 2-amino-8-oxo-9,10-epoxydecanoic acid (AOE). Their epoxy ketone moiety reacts with the target enzyme in an irreversible manner and replacement of the epoxy ketone moiety with $CH_2=CH_2$, CH_2CH_3, or CH_2CH_2OH inhibits HDAC enzyme activity (Ciuffetti et al., 1983; Kijima et al., 1993). Apicidin, a fugal metabolite, belongs to the family of cyclic tetrapeptides; however, it lacks the terminal α-keto-epoxide and thereby it acts as a reversible HDAC inhibitor, and it is important for inhibition of HDAC1 (Darkin-Rattray et al., 1996). Apicidin has potent effects as an anti-proliferating agent against glioblastoma as it induces the tumor suppressor p21Waf1/Cip1 and also gelsolin, which regulate cell cycle and differentiation (Kamitani et al., 2002). Apicidin also shows anti-proliferative activity against various cancer cell lines through selective induction of genes that play important roles in the cell cycle and cell morphology (Han et al., 2000). Bicyclic depsipeptides belong to the second subfamily of cyclic peptides. FK-228, which is the best-studied bicyclic depsipeptide, has been isolated from *Chromobacterium violaceum* and it is capable of inhibiting the growth and progression of tumor cells (Ueda et al., 1994). FK-228 is a stable prodrug that can be activated intracellularly by glutathione reductase by reduction of the disulfide bond to reveal a butenyl thiol moiety, which interacts with Zn^{2+} at the active site of HDAC (Furumai et al., 2002). FK-228 induces apoptosis in human glioblastoma T98G, U251, and U87MG cell lines by decreasing the expression of the anti-apoptotic Bcl-2 and Bcl-xL proteins and increasing the expression of the cell cycle inhibitor p21Waf1/Cip1 (Sawa et al., 2004).

Benzamides, another group of HDAC inhibitors, have shown inhibitory activity against various cancers (Mottamal et al., 2015). Etinostat and Mocetinostat, which are benzamides, are generally active in inhibiting HDAC2 while RG2833 and RGFP966, which are also benzamides, preferably inhibit HDAC3 (Falkenberg and Johnstone, 2014). Entinostat (also known as MS-275) has been shown to be a promising drug against four glioblastoma cell lines (U87MG, C6, F98, and SMA-560) due to induction of cell cycle arrest and apoptotic cell death (Eyüpoglu et al., 2006). Moreover, Entinostat reduces expression of cFLIP(L) and cFLIP(S), which otherwise block the death receptor tumor necrosis factor-related apoptosis-inducing ligand (TRAIL), leading to decreases in recruitment of cFLIP(L) and cFLIP(S) to the TRAIL death-inducing signaling complex and increases in activation of caspase-8 for apoptosis and mitochondria-dependent activation of caspase-9 and -3 for apoptosis in glioblastoma cells (Bangert et al., 2012). Mocetinostast suppress the growth of colon cancer cells by upregulation of Wnt ligand DKK-1 expression (Sikandar et al., 2010) and it induces apoptosis in B-cell chronic lymphocytic leukemia cells by down regulating anti-apoptotic Mcl-1 protein and upregulating pro-apoptotic Bax protein (El-Khoury et al., 2010). But there are no reports yet about the anti-tumor effect of Mocetinostat in glioblastoma. HDAC inhibitors are not only able to target histone but also non-histone proteins that act as HDAC substrate such as transcription factors (e.g., E2F, p53, c-Myc, NF-κB), hypoxia inducible factor-1 alpha (HIF-1α), estrogen receptor alpha (ERα), androgen receptor (AR), myoD chaperone HSP90, and signaling mediators (e.g., Stats, Smad7) (Singh et al., 2010).

Use of these compounds in the biomedical field may represent a new turn in the history of medicine for the treatment of different cancers. The mechanisms and results described above from the studies of the HDAC inhibitors indicate that HDAC inhibitors can be ideal agents for targeting the epigenetic machinery for regulating gene expression in the treatment of many cancers including glioblastoma (Ropero and Esteller, 2007).

SAHA as a Promising Anti-Tumor Agent

SAHA (also known as Vorinostat) is an important pan-HDAC inhibitor that has shown very promising anti-tumor effects in a variety of malignancies due to its high ability to induce differentiation, arrest cell growth, and induce apoptosis (Ugur et al., 2007). SAHA is a linear hydroxamic acid derivative with small molecular weight, it has inhibitory activity against class I (HDAC1, -2, and -3) and class II HDAC enzymes, and it shows wide biological effects in many cancer cell lines (Marks et al., 2001; Ricon, 2006). It has been widely used in clinical trials for cancer therapies (Kelly et al., 2003). This drug has been approved by the US FDA since October 2006 for the treatment of cutaneous T cell lymphoma (Mark, 2007). The discovery of SAHA began 30 years ago when it was found that hexamethylene bisacetmide (HMBA) showed potent effect in induction of growth arrest and differentiation in cancer cells (Mark, 1987). SAHA is more effective than HMBA in inducing growth arrest and differentiation in cancer cells (Richon et al., 1996). There are many reports regarding the role of SAHA in accumulation of acetylate in histone proteins and also non-histone proteins (Figure 2) that regulate many cellular activities including growth and apoptosis (Johnstone and Licht, 2003). Therapeutic efficacy of SAHA has been initially recognized due to its ability to stimulate differentiation in murine erythroleukemia cells in culture and later studies used SAHA in cancer treatments to show its high potential to inhibit tumor growth in rodents (Munster et al., 2001). SAHA significantly contributed to suppression of proliferation of tumor cells and stimulation of differentiation and apoptosis in a variety cancer cells such as breast cancer (Huang and Pardee, 2000), prostate cancer (Lakshmikanthan et al., 2006), non-small cell lung cancer (Feng et al., 2016), glioblastoma (Chiao et al., 2013), pancreatic cancer (Wu et al., 2017), and hepatoma (Wang et al., 2013) cells. Moreover, SAHA has been demonstrated to have high effectiveness in suppression of tumorigenesis in glioblastoma but it triggers autophagy in GSC (Chiao et al., 2013).

Crystallographic studies have demonstrated that the hydroxamic end of SAHA molecule binds to the Zn^{2+} at catalytic pocket of HDAC enzyme and the insertion of the inhibitor SAHA into active site prevents natural substrate from binding, thereby inhibiting deacetylation and leading to accumulation of hyper acetylated histones and acetylated proteins inducing gene transcription. The anti-tumor mechanisms of SAHA are not completely understood yet, but it targets multi-proteins whose acetylation changes their functions in gene expression, cell proliferation, and cell death (Richon, 2006). The glutamate transporter xCT plays a crucial role in progression of glioblastoma, SAHA specifically inhibits the xCT expression, and SAHA dependent xCT reduction is associated with inhibition of ATF4 expression that fosters xCT expression, causing increase in oxidative stress in glioblastoma cells (Wolf et al., 2014).

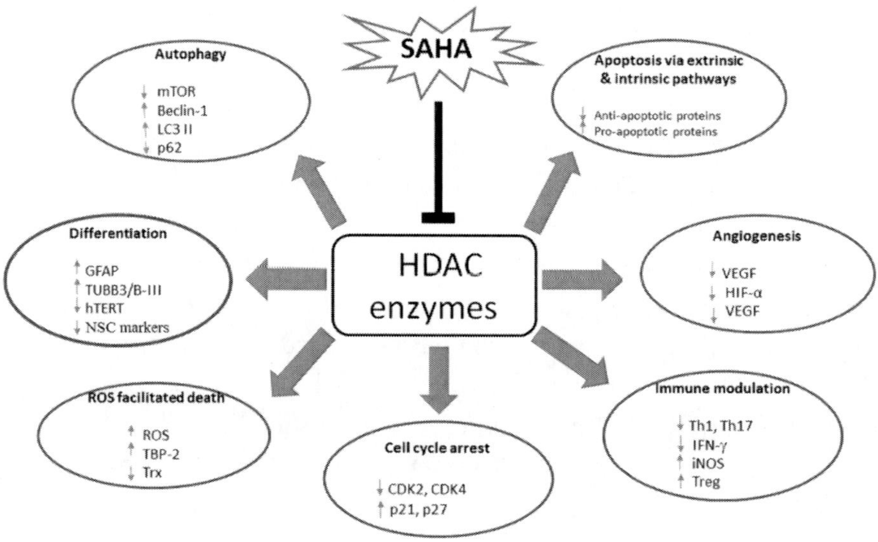

Figure 2. SAHA in regulation of HADC enzymes in glioblastoma cells for controlling autophagy, differentiation, ROS production, apoptosis, cell cycle, angiogenesis, and immune modulation.

Additionally, SAHA plays essential roles in regulation of expression of non-histone proteins (Figure 2) including decrease in expression of deacylated α-tubulin involved in mitosis and the movement of chromosomes via inhibition of HADC6 induced deacylation of α-tubulin (Namdar et al., 2010). SAHA also promotes accumulation of ROS to facilitate cell death in the transformed cells, but not in normal cells, through increase in expression of TBP-2 to reduce thioredoxin (Trx) activity, which contributes to removal of ROS from cancer cells, binding of TBP-2 to Trx activates ASK1 for apoptosis (Butler et al., 2000; Mark et al., 2001). Moreover, SAHA triggers anti-angiogenesis in tumor by repression of transcriptional activity of HIF-1α and vascular endothelial cell factor (VEGF) induced angiogenesis due to inhibition of HDAC family (Hutt et al., 2014). Also, SAHA has important role in inhibition of expression of integrin beta 5, which promotes tumorigenic potential in cancer cells. Integrins significantly contribute to induction of TGF-β activated epithelial-mesenchymal transition (EMT) (Spalletta et al., 2013).

Further, SAHA is one of the important immunomodulatory drugs that play crucial roles in regulation of the host immunity and treatment of immune disorders (Licciardi and Karagiannis, 2012). SAHA has major effects on suppression of Th1 and Th17 cytokines (IL-12 and IL-23, respectively), excretion and activation of dendritic cells (DC), inhibition of chemokines (CXCL9, -10, and -11) (Bosisio et al., 2008). Also, SAHA demonstrated strong roles in controlling immune system by suppression of IL-2 gene expression by the activated T cells and it reduced CD154 (CD40L) and CD25 expression but not CD69 expression (Skov et al., 2003). SAHA has the capability of protection against cytokine-induced toxicity by reduction of expression of the cytokines IFN-γ and IL-1β that are involved in decrease in insulin secretion and increase in inducible nitric oxide synthase (iNOS) to mediate chronic inflammation by macrophages (Larsen et al., 2007). SAHA can upregulate the T regulatory (Treg) cells by activating the expression of CTLA-4 (cytotoxic T lymphocyte-associated protein 4) without affecting T effector cell proliferation and by selectively promoting apoptosis in T effector cells (Zhang et al., 2012).

SAHA as a Double-Edged Sword for Autophagy in Glioblastoma

Autophagy is an ancient Greek word meaning self-eating (El-Bounkari and Bernhagen, 2012) and it is a cellular bulk catabolic process for clearance of damaged mitochondria and other organelles, spoiled and excessive intracellular proteins, and also pathogens by engulfing for digestion with the involvement of lysosome (Glick et al., 2010). Autophagy process begins with formation of double membrane vesicles around the damaged proteins or organelles leading to generation of autophagosomes, which fuse with lysosome to degrade their contents (Suzuki and Ohsumi, 2007). Autophagy is one of the most interesting subjects in cancer research because it is capable of performing quite opposite tasks, cell survival and cell death, depending on the context (Furuya et al., 2004). The role of autophagy in tumor cells is a double-edged sword because it acts as either tumor suppressor or promoter of tumorigenesis in many tissues in the body (Levine and Kroemer, 2008; White, 2012). For tumor suppression, Beclin-1 is overexpressed in normal cells for induction of autophagy to inhibit tumorigenesis by preventing accumulation of the damaged proteins and organelles such as damaged mitochondria, thereby clearing the cells containing toxic oxygen free radicals that cause DNA damage and genomic instability (Brech et al., 2009). Therefore, a reduction in autophagic activity in normal cells may induce tumor growth (Abedin et al., 2007). When Beclin-1 is a heterozygous mutant (Becn1+/-) or Atg5 is down regulated in some cancer cells, autophagy is defective leading to accumulations of p62/SQSTM1, protein aggregates, and damaged mitochondria that result in increase in ROS inside cells leading to DNA damage, genomic instability, and initiation and progression of cancer. Down regulation of p62/SQSTM1 in autophagy-defective cells can inhibit ROS and suppress formation of tumor (Degenhardt et al., 2006; Mathew et al., 2009). Moreover, necrosis and chronic inflammation are also inhibited by autophagy, which thus protects cells against both formation of tumor and acceleration of tumorigenesis (Tang et al., 2010).

On the other hand, autophagy can also act as a tumor promoter when it disturbs and accelerates tumorigenesis. The role of autophagy in tumor development is associated with resistance of tumor cells to stress conditions such as hypoxia and nutrient deprivation. In addition, autophagy can induce ATP production and maintain cellular biosynthesis and survival of tumor cells that use autophagy to provide energy source in episodes of starvation and cellular stress for survival and growth of cells causing progression of tumor (Yang et al., 2011). Also, autophagy may happen because of mutation in the class I phosphoinositide-3-kinase (PI3K) signaling pathway that activates Ras expression to induce autophagy mediated tumorigenesis (Guo et al., 2011). Accumulation of p62/SQSTM1 and damaged mitochondria leading to production of ROS can cause damage to DNA helping tumor progression (White, 2012). Autophagy also induces cancer progression by inhibiting p53 activation that is otherwise involved in autophagy inhibition and this causes growth, invasion, and metastasis of cancer; therefore, cancer cells need autophagy to maintain their survival and progressive growth (White, 2016).

Inhibition of autophagy can lead to suppression of tumor development and its progressive growth (Mazure and Pouyssegur, 2010). So, targeting autophagy in cancer cells is considered an opportunity for treatment of cancer (Yang et al., 2011). However, autophagy is also important in suppression of tumor and activation of autophagy may be a novel strategy for tumor treatment. HDAC inhibitors can play important role in induction of autophagy (Robert et al., 2011) as many studies have demonstrated that HDAC inhibitors have high effectiveness in promoting autophagic cell death in cancer cells (Rikiishi, 2011). SAHA as a pan-HDAC inhibitor is considered to be a potent activator of autophagy (Figure 2) and caspase-dependent apoptotic death in cancer cell lines by upregulating LC3 II and down regulation of Akt/mTOR signaling pathway and stimulation of endoplasmic reticulum stress response causing cell death (Liu et al., 2010).

Recent studies of the ultra-structure of GSC treated with SAHA showed that SAHA suppressed cell growth by inducing excessive autophagy in GSC due to activation of a group of autophagy related factors such as BECN1, LC3 II, and ATG5 and down regulation of Akt/mTOR signaling. Furthermore, SAHA can increase caspase-3 and cleaved poly(ADP-ribose) polymerase (PARP) and reduce accumulation of p62/SQSTM1 that is considered an important inhibitor in autophagy (Chiao et al., 2013). Similar results from other studies have found that SAHA can induce autophagy through accumulation of autophagic factor LC3 II and ULK1 complex, which are considered necessary in inducing autophagy in mouse embryonic fibroblast (MEF) cells, and through down regulation of the nutrient sensing kinase mTOR expression and lysosomal degradation of autophagy substrate (p62/SQSTM1); the same study has also demonstrated that SAHA treatment in glioblastoma T98G cell line stimulates autophagy activation via increase in LC3 II and dramatic decrease in p62/SQSTM1 level (Gammoh et al., 2012). Another study used SAHA with other inhibitors to induce apoptosis, autophagy, or necrosis and found increase in LC3 II level and decrease in p62/SQSTM1 level for autophagy after the glioblastoma GS102 cell line was treated with SAHA and LBH589 combined with oncolytic adenovirus Delta-24-RGD, and thus this could be considered a promising combination therapeutic strategy for treatment of glioblastoma (Berghauser Pont, et al., 2015). On the other hand, SAHA plays critical role in induction of autophagy in glioblastoma cells by inducing lysosome mediated degradation of autophagy substrate p62/SQSTM1 when SAHA was used with BafA1 (Chaio et al., 2013) or down regulation of expression of autophagy proteins such as Beclin-1 and ATG7 when SAHA was used in combination with the caspase inhibitor z-VAD and siRNA (Gammoh et al., 2012). Obviously, SAHA can be considered for inducing non-apoptotic cell death in the tumor cells.

SAHA for Induction of Differentiation in Glioblastoma

Differentiation is a process that turns unspecialized cells to more specialized cells during embryonic development and adult life to perform specific functions in the body. In cancer cells, this process is reversed and thus cancer cells lack differentiation (Jögi et al., 2012). One of the important strategies for anti-tumor therapy is induction of differentiation to make tumor cells mimic normal cells (Takahashi, 2002). Induction of differentiation subsequently could aid induction of apoptosis in human glioblastoma cells in pre-clinical models, as we reported from our studies (Das et al., 2008; Karmakar et al., 2008; Zhang et al., 2008). Induction of HDAC plays important roles in dedifferentiation in cancer cells and HDAC inhibitors significantly contribute to block cell proliferation and overexpression of differentiation genes by increasing accumulation of histone acetylation that leads to conversion of cancer cells to normal cells (Glozak and Seto, 2007). SAHA belongs to the class of HDAC inhibitors that are potent inducer to differentiation (Figure 2) at micromolar or lower concentrations in many types of cancer cells (Marks et al., 2001). Studies showed significant roles for SAHA in induction of differentiation in human breast cancer MCF-7 cell line by arresting cell cycle at G1 and then G2/M phase and by increasing the differentiation markers such as of milk fat globule protein, milk fat membrane globule protein, and lipid droplets; further, SAHA induced differentiation in the estrogen receptor-negative breast cancer SKBR-3 cell line and the retinoblastoma-negative breast cancer MDA-468 cell line (Munster et al., 2001). A later study showed a role for SAHA in induction of differentiation in glioblastoma cells (Chiao et al., 2013). SAHA has high capability of stimulating differentiation in human GSC. SAHA at a dose of 25 μM upregulated expression of differentiation proteins TUBB3/B-III tubulin and GFAP while it down regulated expression of the human telomerase reverse transcriptase (hTERT) and the neural stem cell (NSC) marker proteins PROM1 and Nestin. Human GSC may harbor many stem cell markers (CD133, EGFR, Nanog, Oligo2, and Nestin) and also Yamanaka factors (KLF4, c-Myc, Oct3/4, and Sox2) that can cause therapy resistance (Ray, 2016). SAHA induced differentiation in human GSC and U87MG cells and suppressed the stemness markers such as CD133, Bmi1, Nanog, and Oct3/4 (Hsu et al., 2016). Also, SAHA changed morphological features of cells including enlargement and flattening of GSC. Moreover, SAHA promotes differentiation in K562, HL60, THP-1, and $CD33^+$ cells (Silva et al., 2013).

SAHA for Inhibition of Cell Proliferation and Angiogenesis and Promotion of Apoptosis in Glioblastoma

SAHA, which is a potent pan-HDAC inhibitor, has been shown to induce cell cycle arrest and apoptosis in glioblastoma (Hsu et al., 2016). SAHA regulates autophagy and it is also known for inhibition of cell proliferation and induction of apoptosis (Figure 3) via both extrinsic and intrinsic pathways by down regulating many genes involved in cell proliferation and upregulating other genes responsible for apoptosis and cell cycle arrest (Peart et al., 2005). Generally, SAHA selectively increases expression of pro-apoptotic members of the Bcl-2 family and decreases expression of anti-apoptotic members of this family (Fandy et al., 2005). In intrinsic pathway of apoptosis, SAHA triggers expression of the BH3-only proteins such as Noxa, Puma, Bik, and Bad that can inhibit Bcl-2 and cause release of mitochondrial cytochrome c into cytoplasm; while in extrinsic pathway, SAHA activates TRAIL and induce caspase-8 that in turn directly and indirectly active caspas-3 leading to apoptosis (Al-Yacoub et al., 2012). Many studies have shown a high capability of SAHA in inhibition of cell growth in glioblastoma. High dose of SAHA suppresses cell proliferation in GSC by down regulating expression of stemness markers (CD133 and the Polycomb group protein Bmi1) that are important factors for self-renewal and stemness maintenance in GSC, and SAHA also upregulates p53 and caspase-8 to promote apoptosis (Hsu et al., 2016). Low concentration of SAHA (1 to 25 μM) can cause cell cycle arrest by decreasing levels of expression of Cyclin B1, CDKs, and PCNA and increasing levels of expression of p21, p53, and p38 (Hsu et al., 2016). SAHA can induce cell cycle arrest at G2/M in human glioblastoma U87MG and T89G cell lines and murine glioblastoma GL26 cell line due to its crucial roles in increasing expression of the anti-proliferative proteins such as DR5, TNF-α, p21Waf1/Cip1, and p27Kip1 that can be involved in cell growth arrest and apoptosis, while it reduces many pro-proliferative proteins such as CDK2, CDK4, Cyclin D1, and Cyclin D2 (Yin et al., 2007). Moreover, SAHA increased accumulation of acetylation on H3 histone for 6-fold induction of p21Waf1/Cip1 (Figure 3) (Yin et al., 2007).

SAHA significantly induces apoptosis and inhibits proliferation, migration, and invasion of rat glioblastoma C6 cells in 2D and 3D assays. When rat glioblastoma C6 and human glioblastoma U87MG and LN18 cells are treated with different concentrations of SAHA, the amount of inhibition of cell growth is increased with high concentration of SAHA, it acts to contribute to inhibit MMP2 and MMP9 expression, and it has significant effects on reorganization of collagen I and IV by increasing cell-cell adhesion and E-cadherin that is an important factor in limiting invasion of glioblastoma cells (An et al., 2010). Also, SAHA reduces cell viability in human glioblastoma U87MG cells by decreasing the insulin-like growth factor-1 (IGF-1) receptor signaling pathway that is involved in growth of cells and inhibition of apoptosis (Dharmadhikari, 2015).

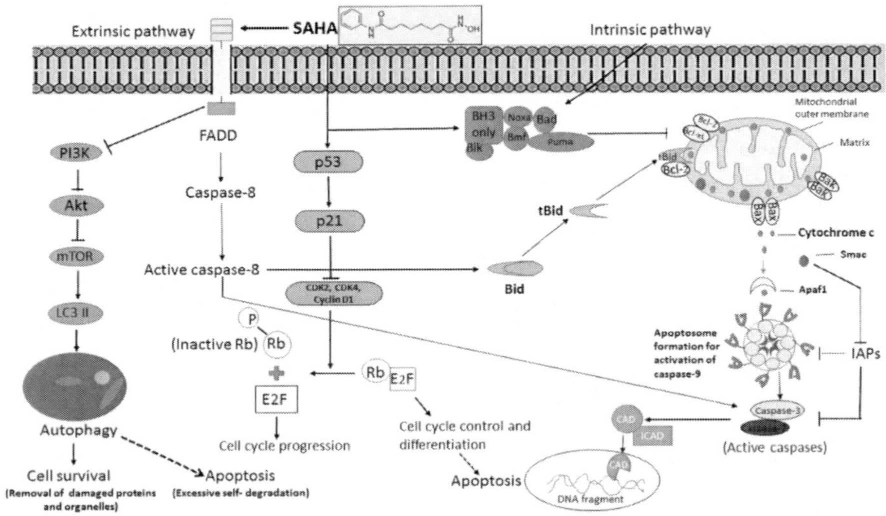

Figure 3. SAHA in modulation of autophagy, cell cycle arrest, induction of differentiation, and activation of the extrinsic and intrinsic pathways of apoptosis in glioblastoma. SAHA may induce limited autophagy for cell survival or excessive autophagy leading to apoptosis. SAHA contributes to cell cycle arrest by inducing p53 that in turn induces p21 to inhibit CDK2, CDK4, and Cyclin D causing binding of Rb to the transcription factor E2F that subsequently induces cell cycle arrest and differentiation. In extrinsic pathway of apoptosis, SAHA induces Fas-associated death domain protein (FADD) to promote cleavage and activation of caspase-8. Active caspase-8 either produces tBid or directly activates caspase-3 and caspase-7 for cleavage of ICAD to release CAD for apoptotic DNA fragmentation. In intrinsic pathway of apoptosis, tBid induces Bax/Bax homo dimerization to cause mitochondrial release of cytochrome c into the cytoplasm. Cytosolic cytochrome c attaches to Apaf1 and forms a complex with pro-caspase-9 (apoptosome). Activation of caspase-9 in turn activates caspase-3 and caspase-7 for apoptosis. Further, SAHA promotes expression of the Bcl-2 homology region 3 (BH3)-only pro-apoptotic proteins such as Bad, Bim, Bid, Noxa, Puma, Bik, and Bmf but inhibition of anti-apoptotic proteins such as Bcl-2 and Bcl-xL or it directly activates the pro-apoptotic multi-BH3 proteins such as Bak and Bax, which induce mitochondrial release of cytochrome c to take apoptotic signaling up to the nucleus for genomic DNA fragmentation.

Enhancer of Zeste 2 (EZH2), the catalytic subunit of Polycomb repressive complex 2 (PRC2), is a histone methyltransferase that targets Lys-27 of histone H3 (H3K27) (Valk-Lingbeek et al., 2004). EZH2 is a key member for the function of PRC2. Chromatin marking by H3K27 can also be relevant in the oncogenesis of glioblastoma. Trimethylated H3K27 (H3K27me3) in chromatin is a common marker of silencing of differentiation genes. EZH2 causes repression of expression of tumor suppressor and promotes growth of GSC. Indeed, EZH2 expression could be significant in GSC in grade IV brain tumor, as reported by a recent study (Orzan et al., 2011). Treatment of GSC with SAHA caused significant upregulation of PRC2 predicted target genes, disrupted proliferation of GSC, and decreased expression of EZH2 and the stemness marker CD133. Inhibition of expression of EZH2 by shRNA was associated with a significant decrease in proliferation of glioblastoma cells. Exposure of GSC from a grade IV brain tumor (GBMR1) to 1, 2, or 5 μM SAHA for 48 h showed dose-dependent decrease in EZH2 expression leading to decrease in proliferation of GSC (Orzan et al., 2011). SAHA inhibited tumor growth in an orthotropic model of glioblastoma, as histological analysis showed that 80% of tumor volume was reduced due to treatment with SAHA and this was associated with reductions in tumor cell growth and also angiogenesis (Ugur et al., 2007). Moreover, SAHA is found to be orally active and it has high efficacy in suppression of tumor growth and no effect on normal brain tissue in rats with orthotopic glioblastoma (Wei et al., 2012). Untreated tumors exhibited significantly increases in alanine and lactate levels and decreases in inositol, N-acetylaspartate, and creatine levels, the typical metabolic markers in glioblastoma relative to normal brain tissues. These metabolites were restored to the levels found in normal-like brain tissues after SAHA treatment of glioblastoma in rats, suggesting that these could be the reliable metabolic biomarkers at the earliest stage of SAHA treatment of glioblastoma to predict the therapeutic response (Wei et al., 2012).

Synergistic Efficacy of SAHA in Combination with Other Anti-Tumor Drugs

Drug synergy is the cooperation between two drugs to increase their therapeutic effectiveness in the treatment of diseases such as cancer, cardiovascular disease, and infectious disease. Also, lessening the doses of two drugs in combination enhance therapeutic effectiveness and avoid side effects (Chou et al., 2006, Karmakar et al., 2009, Mohan et al., 2011). The main principle of combination therapy is targeting different signaling pathways or multi-mechanisms in the cells or pathogen to decrease the chance of resistance to the therapy by the cells or organism (Mohan et al., 2013; Bansal et al., 2014). Results reported from our laboratory showed that synergism of two anti-tumor agents could dramatically increase therapeutic efficacy in different rat glioblastoma cell lines (Janardhanan et al., 2009) and human glioblastoma cell lines as well as in GSC (Hossain et al., 2012; Chakrabarti and Ray, 2015). There are many HDAC inhibitors nowadays for treatment of cancer cells (Choi et al., 2011). These HDAC inhibitors have important roles in inhibition of tumor growth but they are still limited to suppression of solid tumor growth when they are used alone (Singh et al., 2015). There are some HDAC inhibitors to suppress specific pathways of cell cycle while other cell survival pathways still remain active. So, two inhibitors in combination may enhance therapeutic effect for blocking tumor cell growth (Liu et al., 2007).

Aggressive development and progression of glioblastoma pushed the interest for identifying specific small molecule inhibitors for treatment of glioblastoma. The small molecule SAHA is a pan-HDAC inhibitor that is a promising therapeutic agent in the treatment of cancer when it is used in combination with another small molecule inhibitor (Kerl et al., 2013). SAHA combined with other inhibitor has a better effect in targeting glioblastoma cells than when it is used alone (Rasmussen et al., 2016). Synergistic effects of SAHA and another anti-tumor agent have been observed in a variety of experiments in the treatment of glioblastoma. One of the studies has shown that glioblastoma cells treated with the retinoid all-*trans* retinoic acid (ATRA) alone was not beneficial in eliminating tumor cells, but combination of ATRA and SAHA significantly contributed to suppression of progressive growth of human stem-like glioblastoma cells (SLGC) and also increased the number of apoptotic cells in the tumor tissue (Schmoch et al., 2016). Other studies have used combination of two different HDAC inhibitors, SAHA and VPA, in inhibiting cell growth in human glioblastoma U251MG and LN299 cells, and found that both HDAC inhibitors together had more inhibitory activities than the conventional chemotherapeutic drug Temozolomide in suppression of glioblastoma cell proliferation and clonogenicity (Cornago et al., 2014). Also, it has been observed that SAHA and VPA can cause increases in production of ROS for apoptosis via mitochondrial pathway in glioblastoma (Cornago et al., 2014). The HADC inhibitor SAHA and the topoisomerase I inhibitor SN38 in combination had more potent cytotoxic effects and superior therapeutic efficacy than SN38 alone suggesting that this combination of drugs contributed to the improvement of efficacy in the treatment of glioblastoma (Sarcar et al., 2010). Administration of combination of SAHA and Olaparib enhanced inhibitory effects in elimination of xenografted glioblastoma cells by induction of apoptosis, because HDAC1 and PARP (a DNA repair enzyme) levels were decreased due to combination treatment; also, DNA double strand breaks were increased to enhance induction of apoptosis when two drugs were used together (Rasmussen et al., 2016).

Expression of the anti-apoptotic Bcl-2 protein was decreased to 90% while the tumor suppressor p53 induced apoptosis was significantly increased when SAHA and 3 Gy RTX were used together in the treatment of glioblastoma GS79 and GS275 cells; SAHA and 3 Gy RTX upregulated p21 to 110% and increased expression of caspase-3 and caspase-7; they contributed to increase in acetylated histone H3; and synergism between SAHA and RTX induced phosphorylation of checkpoint kinase 2 (pCHEK2) that could mediate DNA damage signaling by phosphorylating and activating p53, blocked cell cycle progression, and induced apoptosis in response to DNA damage (Berghauser Pont et al., 2015).

Another investigation identified a new strategy to increase efficacy of SAHA by its combination with tranylcypromine, an inhibitor for another epigenetic enzyme LSD1/KDM1A (lysine-specific demethylase 1), for controlling growth of human glioblastoma LN18 and U87MG cells with induction of apoptotic cell death in vitro and in vivo (Singh et al., 2015). Interestingly, a recent study showed that SAHA could play a critical role in promoting hyper radio sensitivity in human glioblastoma D54 cells (p53 and PTEN wild type) and U118 cells (p53 and PTEN mutants), as the data indicated that cells were killed when treated with the combination of SAHA and radiation by activation of caspase-3 (Diss et al., 2014). The Bcl-2 inhibitor ABT-737, an anti-tumor drug, failed in inhibiting proliferation of glioblastoma cells when it was used alone but combination of SAHA and ABT-737 dramatically led to induction of apoptosis by increasing pro-apoptotic proteins Noxa, tBid, and Bax (Foster et al., 2014). Combination of these anti-tumor drugs, SAHA and ABT-737, enhanced cell death via inactivation of the PI3K/Akt survival signaling pathway and sensitization of the PTEN-deleted glioblastoma cells (Foster et al., 2014).

CONCLUSION

In conclusion, HDAC enzymes are epigenetic modulators of gene expression that can cause tumors by inhibiting expression of proteins that induce cell cycle arrest, differentiation, and apoptosis. HDAC inhibitors are the new anti-tumor drugs for promotion of acetylation of histone and non-histone proteins for transcription of several genes for cell death. We previously reported that combination of one HDAC inhibitor and another anti-tumor drug could work synergistically for controlling growth of human glioblastoma cells (Roy Choudhury et al., 2011). Recent studies from our laboratories also strongly suggest that HDAC inhibition is an important therapeutic strategy for prevention of tumor growth progression and promotion of apoptosis in animal model of glioblastoma (Wallace et al., 2013). SAHA is a pan-HDAC inhibitor that has been approved by the US FDA for treatment of T cell lymphoma and it has anti-tumor effects in glioblastoma cell lines in vitro and in vivo as it is effective in inducing differentiation and apoptosis but suppressing growth arrest and angiogenesis. SAHA can increase the acetylation in the core histones H3 and H4 and down regulate anti-apoptotic Bcl-2 protein and upregulate pro-apoptotic Bax protein. Also, SAHA plays a major role in modulation of autophagy and it may inhibit autophagy in tumor cells when it is used in combination with another inhibitor. The synergism between SAHA and another anti-tumor drug can lead to increase in their therapeutic efficiency for induction of differentiation and apoptosis in human glioblastoma cells.

ACKNOWLEDGMENTS

This work was supported in part by an incentive award from the Soy Health Research Program (SHRP, United Soybean Board, Chesterfield, MO, US), the Investigator Initiated Research grant (SCIRF-2015-I-0) from the State of South Carolina Spinal Cord Injury Research Fund (SCIRF, Columbia, SC, US), and also the previously awarded R01 grants (CA91460 and NS057811) from the National Institutes of Health (Bethesda, MD, US) to SKR.

REFERENCES

Abbas A, Gupta S (2008) Role histone deacetylase in prostate cancer. *Epigenetics* 3:300-309.

Abedin MJ, Wang D, McDonnell MA, Lehmann U, Kelekar A (2007) Autophagy delays apoptotic death in breast cancer cells following DNA damage. *Cell Death Differ* 14:500-510.

Adom D, Nie D (2013) Regulation of autophagy by short chain fatty acids in colon cancer cells. In: *Autophagy - A Double-Edged Sword - Cell Survival or Death?* (Bailly Y, editor), In Tech, Rijeka, Croatia, p. 235-247.

Al-Yacoub N, Fecker LF, Möbs M, Plötz M, Braun FK, Sterry W, Eberle J (2012) Apoptosis induction by SAHA in cutaneous T-cell lymphoma cells is related to downregulation of c-FLIP and enhanced TRAIL signaling. *J Invest Dermatol* 9:2263-2274.

An Z, Gluck CB, Choy ML, Kaufman LJ (2010) Suberoylanilide hydroxamic acid limits migration and invasion of glioma cells in two and three-dimensional culture. *Cancer Lett* 292:215-227.

Andriamihaja M, Chaumontet C, Tome D (2009) Butyrate metabolism in human colon carcinoma cells: Implications concerning its growth-inhibitory effect. *J Cell Physiol* 218: 58-65.

Appin CL, Brat DJ (2015) Molecular pathways in gliomagenesis and their relevance to neuropathologic diagnosis. *Adv Anat Pathol* 22:50-58.

Banelli B, Carra E, Barbieri F, Würth R, Parodi F, Pattarozzi A, Carosio R, Forlani A, Allemanni G, Marubbi D, Florio T, Daga A, Romani M (2015) The histone demethylase KDM5A is a key factor for the resistance to temozolomide in glioblastoma. *Cell Cycle* 14:3418-3429.

Bangert A, Cristofanon S, Eckhardt I, Abhari BA, Kolodziej S, Häcker S, Vellanki SH, Lausen J, Debatin KM, Fulda S (2012) Histone deacetylase inhibitors sensitize glioblastoma cells to TRAIL-induced apoptosis by c-Myc-mediated downregulation of cFLIP. *Oncogene* 31:4677-4688.

Bansal M, Yang J, Karan C, Menden MP, Costello JC, Tang H, Xiao C, Li Y (2014) A community computational challenge to predict the activity of pairs of compounds. *Nat Biotechnol* 32:1213-1222.

Berendsen S, Broekman M, Seute T, Snijders T, Van Es C, de Vos F, Regli L, Robe P (2012) Valproic acid for the treatment of malignant gliomas: review of the preclinical rationale and published clinical results. *Expert Opin Investig Drugs* 21:1391-1415.

Berghauser Pont LM, Kleijn A, Kloezeman JJ, van den Bossche W, Kaufmann JK, de Vrij J, Leenstra S, Dirven CM, Lamfers ML (2015) The HDAC inhibitors Scriptaid and LBH589 combined with the oncolytic virus Delta24-RGD exert enhanced anti-tumor efficacy in patient-derived glioblastoma cells. *PLoS One* 10:e0127058.

Bertos NR, Wang AH, Yang XJ (2001) Class II histone deacetylases: structure, function and regulation. *Biochem Cell Biol* 79:243-252.

Bezecny P (2014) Histone deacetylase inhibitors in glioblastoma: pre-clinical and clinical experience. *Med Oncol* 31:985.

Bischof J, Westhoff MA, Wagner JE, Halatsch ME, Trentmann S, Knippschild U, Wirtz CR, Burster T (2017) Cancer stem cells: The potential role of autophagy, proteolysis, and cathepsins in glioblastoma stem cells. *Tumour Biol* 39:1010428317692227.

Bondy ML, Scheurer ME, Malmer B, Barnholtz-Sloan JS, Davis FG, Il'yasova D, Kruchko C, McCarthy BJ, Rajaraman P, Schwartzbaum JA, Sadetzki S, Schlehofer B, Tihan T, Wiemels JL, Wrensch M, Buffler PA; Brain Tumor Epidemiology Consortium (2008) Brain tumor epidemiology: Consensus from the Brain Tumor Epidemiology Consortium. *Cancer* 113:1953-1968.

Boosalis MS, Bandyopadhyay R, Bresnick EH (2001) Short-chain fatty acid derivatives stimulate cell proliferation and induce STAT-5 activation. *Blood* 97:3259-3267.

Bosisio D, Vulcano M, Del Prete A, Sironi M, Slave V (2008) Blocking TH17-polarizing cytokines by histone deacetylase inhibitors in vitro and in vivo. *J Leuk Biol* 84:1540-1548.

Brech A, Ahlquist T, Lothe RA, Stenmark A (2009) Autophagy in tumor suppression and promotion. *Mol Oncol* 3:366-375.

Bukowska B, Gajek A, Marczak A (2015) Two drugs are better than one. A short history of combined therapy of ovarian cancer. *Contemp Oncol* 19:350-353.

Butler LM, Agus DB, Scher, HI, Higgins B, Rose A, Cordon-Cardo C, Thaler HT, Rifkind RA, Marks PA, Richon VM (2000) Suberoylanilide hydroxamic acid, an inhibitor of histone deacetylase, suppresses the growth of prostate cancer cells in vitro and in vivo. *Cancer Res* 60:5165-5170.

Campos B, Bermejo JL, Han L, Felsberg J, Ahmadi R, Grabe N, Reifenberger G, Unterberg A, Herold-Mende C (2011) Expression of nuclear receptor corepressors and class I histone deacetylases in astrocytic gliomas. *Cancer Sci* 102:387-392.

Carew JS, Giles FJ, Nawrocki ST (2008) Histone deacetylase inhibitors: mechanisms of cell death and promise in combination cancer therapy. *Cancer Lett* 269:07-17.

Chakrabarti M, Banik NL, Ray SK (2013) Photofrin based photodynamic therapy and miR-99a transfection inhibited FGFR3 and PI3K/Akt signaling mechanisms to control growth of human glioblastoma in vitro and in vivo. *PLoS One* 8:e55652.

Chakrabarti M, Klionsky DJ, Ray SK (2016) miR-30e Blocks autophagy and acts synergistically with proanthocyanidin for inhibition of AVEN and BIRC6 to increase apoptosis in glioblastoma stem cells and glioblastoma SNB19 Cells. *PLoS One* 11:e0158537.

Chakrabarti M, Ray SK (2015) Synergistic anti-tumor actions of luteolin and silibinin prevented cell migration and invasion and induced apoptosis in glioblastoma SNB19 cells and glioblastoma stem cells. *Brain Res* 1629:85-93.

Chen HP, Zhao YT, Zhao T (2015) Histone deacetylases and mechanisms of regulation of gene expression (histone deacetylases in cancer). *Crit Rev Oncog* 20:35-47.

Chiao MT, Cheng WY, Yang YC, Shen CC, Ko JL (2013) Suberoylanilide hydroxamic acid (SAHA) causes tumor growth slowdown and triggers autophagy in glioblastoma stem cells. *Autophagy* 10:1509-1526.

Choi E, Lee C, Park JE, Seo JJ, Cho M, Kang JS, Kim HM, Park SK, Lee K, Han G (2011) Structure and property based design, synthesis and biological evaluation of γ-lactam based HDAC inhibitors. *Bioorg Med Chem Lett* 21:1218-1221.

Chou TC (2006) Theoretical basis, experimental design, and computerized simulation of synergism and antagonism in drug combination studies. *Pharmacol Rev* 58:621-681.

Ciuffetti LM, Pope MR, Dunkle LD, Daly JM, Knoche HW (1983) Isolation and structure of an inactive product derived from the host-specific toxin produced by *Helminthosporium carbonum*. *Biochemistry* 22:3507-3510.

Coffey DC, Kutko MC, Glick RD, Butler LM, Heller G, Rifkind RA, Marks PA, Richon VM, La Quaglia MP (2001) The histone deacetylase inhibitor, CBHA, inhibits growth of human neuroblastoma xenografts in vivo, alone and synergistically with all-*trans* retinoic acid. *Cancer Res* 61:3591-3594.

Cornago M, Garcia-Alberich C, Blasco-Angulo N, Vall-Llaura N, Nager M, Herreros, J Comella JX, Sanchis D, Llovera M (2014) Histone deacetylase inhibitors promote glioma cell death by G2 checkpoint abrogation leading to mitotic catastrophe. *Cell Death Dis* 5:e1435.

Darkin-Rattray SJ, Gurnett AM, Myers RW, Dulski PM, Crumley TM, Allocco JJ, Cannova C, Meinke PT, Colletti SL, Bednarek MA, Singh SB, Goetz MA, Dombrowski AW, Polishook JD, Schmatz DM (1996) Apicidin A novel antiprotozoal agent that inhibits parasite histone deacetylase. *Proc Natl Acad Sci USA* 93:13143-13147.

Das A, Banik NL, Ray SK (2008) Retinoids induced astrocytic differentiation with down regulation of telomerase activity and enhanced sensitivity to taxol for apoptosis in human glioblastoma T98G and U87MG cells. *J Neuro-oncol* 87:9-22.

De Ruijter AJM, van Gennip AH, Caron HN, Kemp S, van Kuilenburg ABP. (2003) Histone deacetylases (HDACs): characterization of the classical HDAC family. *Biochem J* 370:737-749.

Degenhardt K, Mathew R, Beaudoin B, Bray K, Anderson D, Chen G, Mukherjee C, Shi Y, Gélinas C, Fan Y, Nelson DA, White E (2006) Autophagy promotes tumor cell survival and restricts necrosis, inflammation, and tumorigenesis. *Cancer Cell* 10:51-64.

Deroanne CF, Bonjean K, Servotte S, Devy L, Colige A, Clausse N, Blacher S, Verdin E, Foidart JM, Nusgens BV, Castronovo V (2002) Histone deacetylases inhibitors as anti-angiogenic agents altering vascular endothelial growth factor signaling. *Oncogene* 21:427-436.

Deubzer HE, Schier MC, Oehme I, Lodrini M, Haendler B, Sommer A, Witt O (2013) HDAC11 is a novel drug target in carcinomas. *Int J Cancer* 132:2200-2208.

Dharmadhikari R (2015) SAHA (Vorinostat) imparts anti-neoplastic effects against glioblastoma multiforme via IGF-1R signaling pathway (Doctoral dissertation), Long Island University, Retrieved from *ProQuest Dissertations and Theses* 1526670.

Di Marcotullio L, Canettieri G, Infante P, Greco A, Gulino A (2011) Protected from the inside: endogenous histone deacetylase inhibitors and the road to cancer. *Biochim Biophys Acta* 1815:241-252.

Diss E, Nalabothula N, Nguyen D, Chang E, Kwok Y, Carrier F (2014) Vorinostat SAHA promotes hyper-radiosensitivity in wild type p53 human glioblastoma cells. *J Clin Oncol Res* 2:1-9.

Drummond DC, Noble CO, Kirpotin DB, Guo Z, Scott GK, Benz CC (2005) Clinical development of histone deacetylase inhibitors as anticancer agents. *Annu Rev Pharmacol Toxicol* 45:495-528.

Duvic M, Vu J (2007) Vorinostat: a new oral histone deacetylase inhibitor approved for cutaneous T-cell lymphoma. *Expert Opin Investig Drugs* 16:1111-1120.

El Bounkari O, Bernhagen J (2012). MIF and autophagy: a novel link beyond "eating." *Cell Res* 22:930-953.

El-Khoury V, Moussay E, Janji B, Palissot V, Aouali N, Brons NH, Van Moer K, Pierson S, Van Dyck E, Berchem G (2010) The histone deacetylase inhibitor MGCD0103 induces apoptosis in B-cell chronic lymphocytic leukemia cells through a mitochondria-mediated caspase activation cascade. *Mol Cancer Ther* 9:1349-1360.

Entin-Meer M, Rephaeli A, Yang X, Nudelman A, VandenBerg SR, Haas-Kogan DA (2005) Butyric acid prodrugs are histone deacetylase inhibitors that show antineoplastic activity and radiosensitizing capacity in the treatment of malignant gliomas. *Mol Cancer Ther* 4:1952-1961.

Eyüpoglu IY, Hahnen E, Buslei R, Siebzehnrübl FA, Savaskan NE, Lüders M, Tränkle C, Wick W, Weller M, Fahlbusch R, Blümcke I (2005) Suberoylanilide hydroxamic acid (SAHA) has potent anti-glioma properties in vitro, ex vivo and in vivo. *J Neurochem* 93:992-999.

Eyüpoglu IY, Hahnen E, Tränkle C, Savaskan NE, Siebzehnrübl FA, Busle I R, Lemke D, Wick W, Fahlbusch R, Blümcke I (2006) Experimental therapy of malignant gliomas using the inhibitor of histone deacetylase MS-275. *Mol Cancer Ther* 5:1248-1255.

Falkenberg KJ, Johnstone RW (2014) Histone deacetylases and their inhibitors in cancer, neurological diseases and immune disorders. *Nat Rev Drug Discov* 13:673-691.

Fandy TE, Shankar S, Ross DD, Sausville E, Srivastava RK (2005) Interactive effects of HDAC inhibitors and TRAIL on apoptosis are associated with changes in mitochondrial functions and expressions of cell cycle regulatory genes in multiple myeloma. *Neoplasia* 7:646-657.

Feng J, Zhang S, Wu K, Wang B, Wong JY, Jiang H, Xu R, Ying L, Huang H, Zheng X, Chen X, Ma S (2016) Combined effects of suberoylanilide hydroxamic acid and cisplatin on radiation sensitivity and cancer cell invasion in non-small cell lung cancer. *Mol Cancer Ther* 15:842-853.

Ferlay J, Steliarova-Foucher E, Lortet-Tieulent J, Rosso S, Coebergh JW, Comber H, Forman D, Bray F (2013) Cancer incidence and mortality patterns in Europe: Estimates for 40 countries in 2012. *Eur J Cancer* 49:1374-1403.

Finnin MS, Donigian JR, Cohen A, Richon VM, Rifkind RA, Marks PA, Breslow R, Pavletich NP (1999) Structures of a histone deacetylase homologue bound to the TSA and SAHA inhibitors. *Nature* 401:188-193.

Foster KA, Jane EP, Premkumar DR, Morales A, Pollack IF (2014) Co-administration of ABT-737 and SAHA induces apoptosis, mediated by Noxa upregulation, Bax activation and mitochondrial dysfunction in PTEN-intact malignant human glioma cell lines. *J Neuro-Oncol* 120:459-472.

Frolov MV, Dyson NJ (2004) Molecular mechanisms of E2F-dependent activation and pRB-mediated repression. *J Cell Sci* 117:2173-2181.

Furumai R, Matsuyama A, Kobashi N, Lee KH, Nishiyama M, Nakajima H, Tanaka A, Komatsu Y, Nishino N, Yoshida M, Horinouchi S (2002) FK228 (depsipeptide) as a natural prodrug that inhibits class I histone deacetylases. *Cancer Res* 62:4916-4921.

Furuya N, Liang XH, Levin B (2004) Autophagy and cancer. In: *Autophagy* (Klionsky DJ, editor), Landes Bioscience, Georgetown, TX, USA, p. 244-253.

Galanis E, Jaeckle KA, Maurer MJ, Reid JM, Ames MM, Hardwick JS, Reilly JF, Loboda A, Nebozhyn M, Fantin VR, Richon VM, Scheithauer B, Giannini C, Flynn PJ, Moore DF Jr, Zwiebel J, Buckner JC (2009) Phase II trial of Vorinostat in recurrent glioblastoma multiforme: a north central cancer treatment group study. *J Clin Oncol* 27:2052-2058.

Gallinari P, Di Marco S, Jones P, Pallaoro M, Steinkühler C (2007) HDACs, histone deacetylation and gene transcription: from molecular biology to cancer therapeutics. *Cell Res* 17:195-211.

Gammoh N, Lam D, Puente C, Ganley I, Marks PA, Jiang X (2012) Role of autophagy in histone deacetylase inhibitor-induced apoptotic and nonapoptotic cell death. *Proc Natl Acad Sci USA* 9:6561-6565.

George J, Banik NL, Ray SK (2009) Combination of taxol and Bcl-2 siRNA induces apoptosis in human glioblastoma cells and inhibits invasion, angiogenesis and tumour growth. *J Cell Mol Med* 13:4205-4218.

George J, Banik NL, Ray SK (2010) Knockdown of hTERT and concurrent treatment with interferon-gamma inhibited proliferation and invasion of human glioblastoma cell lines. *Int J Biochem Cell Biol* 42:1164-1173.

George J, Banik NL, Ray SK (2010) Survivin knockdown and concurrent 4-HPR treatment controlled human glioblastoma in vitro and in vivo. *Neuro Oncol* 12:1088-1101.

Gilbert KM, DeLoose A, Valentine JL, Fifer EK (2006) Structure–activity relationship between carboxylic acids and T cell cycle blockade. *Life Sci* 78:2159-2165.

Glick D, Barth S, Macleod KF (2010) Autophagy: cellular and molecular mechanisms. *J Pathol* 221:3-12.

Glozak MA, Sengupta N, Zhang X, Seto E. (2005). Acetylation and deacetylation of non-histone proteins. *Gene* 363:15-23.

Glozak MA, Seto E (2007) Histone deacetylases and cancer. *Oncogene* 26:5420-5432.

Goussia AC, Agnantis NJ, Rao JS, Kyritsis AP (2000) Cytogenetic and molecular abnormalities in astrocytic gliomas. *Oncol Rep* 2:401-412.

Gregoretti IV, Lee YM, Goodson HV (2004) Molecular evolution of the histone deacetylase family: functional implications of phylogenetic analysis. *J Mol Biol* 338:17-31.

Guan JS, Haggarty SJ, Giacometti E, Dannenberg JH, Joseph N, Gao J, Nieland TJ, Zhou Y, Wang X, Mazitschek R, Bradner JE, DePinho RA, Jaenisch R and Tsai, LH (2009) HDAC2 negatively regulates memory formation and synaptic plasticity. *Nature* 459:55-60.

Gui CY, Ngo L, Xu WS, Richon VM, Marks PA (2004) Histone deacetylase (HDAC) inhibitor activation of p21Waf1 involves changes in promoter-associated proteins, including HDAC1. *Proc Natl Acad Sci USA* 101:1241-1246.

Guo JY, Chen HY, Mathew R, Fan J, Strohecker AM, Karsli-Uzunbas G, Kamphorst JJ, Chen G, Lemons JM, Karantza V, Coller HA, Dipaola RS, Gelinas C, Rabinowitz JD, White E (2011) Activated Ras requires autophagy to maintain oxidative metabolism and tumorigenesis. *Genes Dev* 25:460-470.

Han JW, Ahn SH, Park SH, Wang SY, Bae GU and Seo, DW (2000) Apicidin, a histone deacetylase inhibitor, inhibits proliferation of tumor cells *via* induction of p21Waf1/Cip1 and gelsolin. *Cancer Res* 60:6068-6074.

He X, Nie H, Hong Y, Sheng C, Xia W and Ying, W (2012) SIRT2 activity is required for the survival of C6 glioma cells. *Biochem Biophys Res Commun* 417:468-472.

Höring E, Podlech O, Silkenstedt B, Rota IA, Adamopoulou E, Naumann U (2013) The histone deacetylase inhibitor Trichostatin A promotes apoptosis and antitumor immunity in glioblastoma cells. *Anticancer Res* 33:1351-1360.

Hossain M, Banik NL, Ray SK (2012) Synergistic anti-cancer mechanisms of curcumin and paclitaxel for growth inhibition of human brain tumor stem cells and LN18 and U138MG cells. *Neurochem Int* 61:1102-1113.

Hsu C, Chang W, Hsu T, Liu J, Yeh S, Wang J, Liou J, Ko C, Chang K, Chuang J (2016) Suberoylanilide hydroxamic acid represses glioma stem-like cells. *J Biomed Sci* 23: 81.

Hu E, Dul E Sung CM, Chen Z, Kirkpatrick R, Zhang GF (2003) Identification of novel isoform-selective inhibitors within class I histone deacetylases. *J Pharmacol Exp Ther* 307:720-728.

Huang BH, Laban M, Leung CH, Lee L, Lee CK, Salto-Tellez M, Raju GC, Hooi SC (2005) Inhibition of histone deacetylase 2 increases apoptosis and p21Cip1/Waf1 expression, independent of histone deacetylase 1. *Cell Death Differ* 12:395-404.

Huang L and Pardee AB (2000) Suberoylanilide hydroxamic acid as a potential therapeutic agent for human breast cancer treatment. *Mol Med* 6:849-866.

Hutt DM, Roth DM, Vignaud H, Cullin C, Bouchecareilh M (2014) The histone deacetylase inhibitor, Vorinostat, represses hypoxia inducible factor 1 alpha expression through translational inhibition. *PLoS One* 9:e106224.

Imaoka N, Hiratsuka M, Osaki M, Kamitani H, Kambe A, Fukuoka J, Kurimoto M, Nagai S, Okada F, Watanabe T, Ohama E, Kato S, Oshimura M (2012) Prognostic significance of sirtuin 2 protein nuclear localization in glioma: an immunohistochemical study. *Oncol Rep* 28:923-930.

Janardhanan R, Banik NL, Ray SK (2008) N-(4-Hydroxyphenyl) retinamide induced differentiation with repression of telomerase and cell cycle to increase interferon-gamma sensitivity for apoptosis in human glioblastoma cells. *Cancer Lett* 261:26-36.

Janardhanan R, Butler JT, Banik NL, Ray SK (2009) N-(4-Hydroxyphenyl) retinamide potentiated paclitaxel for cell cycle arrest and apoptosis in glioblastoma C6 and RG2 cells. *Brain Res* 1268:142-153.

Jögi A, Vaapil M, Johansson M, Påhlman S (2012) Cancer cell differentiation heterogeneity and aggressive behavior in solid tumors. *Ups J Med Sci* 117:217-224.

Johnstone RW, Licht JD (2003) Histone deacetylase inhibitors in cancer therapy: is transcription the primary target. *Cancer Cell* 4:13–18.

Jones P (2009) Histone deacetylase inhibitors. In: *Epigenetic Targets in Drug Discovery* (Sippl W, Jung M, editors), Vol. 42, Wiley-VCH, Weinheim, Germany, p.185-223.

Juan LJ, Shia WJ, Chen MH, Yang WM, Seto E, Lin YS, Wu CW (2000) Histone deacetylases specifically down-regulate p53-dependent gene activation. *J Biol Chem* 275:20436-20443.

Jung KH, Noh JH, Kim JK, Eun JW, Bae HJ, Xie HJ, Chang YG, Kim MG, Park H, Lee JY, Nam SW (2012) HDAC2 overexpression confers oncogenic potential to human lung cancer cells by deregulating expression of apoptosis and cell cycle proteins. *J Cell Biochem* 113:2167-2177.

Kamitani H, Taniura S, Watanabe K, Sakamoto M, Watanabe T, Eling T (2002) Histone acetylation may suppress human glioma cell proliferation when p21Waf1/Cip1 and gelsolin are induced. *Neuro Oncol* 4:95-101.

Karagianni P, Wong J (2007). HDAC3: taking the SMRT-N-CoRrect road to repression. *Oncogene* 26:5439-5449.

Karmakar S, Banik NL, Ray SK (2008) Combination of all-*trans* retinoic acid and paclitaxel induced differentiation and apoptosis in human glioblastoma U87MG xenografts in nude mice. *Cancer* 112:596-607.

Karmakar S, Choudhury SR, Banik NL, Ray SK (2009) Combination of N-(4-hydroxyphenyl) retinamide and genistein increased apoptosis in neuroblastoma SK-N-BE2 and SH-SY5Y xenografts. *Neuroscience* 163:286-295.

Kelly WK, Richon VM, O'Connor O, Curley T, MacGregor-Curtelli B, Tong W, Klang M, Schwartz L, Richardson S, Rosa E, Drobnjak M, Cordon-Cordo C, Chiao JH, Rifkind R, Marks, PA and Scher H (2003) Phase I clinical trial of histone deacetylase inhibitor: suberoylanilide hydroxamic acid administered intravenously. *Clin Cancer Res* 1:3578-3588.

Kerl K, Ries D, Unland R, Borchert C, Moreno N, Hasselblatt M, Jürgens H, Kool M, Görlich D, Eveslage M, Jung M, Meisterernst M, Frühwald M (2013) The histone deacetylase inhibitor SAHA acts in synergism with fenretinide and doxorubicin to control growth of rhabdoid tumor cells. *BMC Cancer* 13:286.

Kijima MY, Oshida M, Sugita K, Horinouchi S, Beppu T (1993) Trapoxin, an antitumor cyclic tetrapeptide, is an irreversible inhibitor of mammalian histone deacetylase. *J Biol Chem* 268:22429-22435.

Kim H, Bae S (2011) Histone deacetylase inhibitors: molecular mechanisms of action and clinical trials as anti-cancer drugs. *Am J Transl Res* 3:166-179.

Komata T, Kanzawa T, Nashimoto T, Aoki H, Endo S, Kon T, Takahashi H, Kondo S, Tanaka R (2005) Histone deacetylase inhibitors, N-butyric acid and trichostatin A, induce caspase-8- but not caspase-9-dependent apoptosis in human malignant glioma cells. *Int J Oncol* 26:1345-1352.

Krex D, Klink B, Hartmann C, von Deimling A, Pietsch T, Simon M, Sabel M, Steinbach JP, Heese O, Reifenberger G, Weller M, Schackert G; German Glioma Network (2007) Long-term survival with glioblastoma multiforme. *Brain* 130:2596-2606.

Kumagai T, Wakimoto N, Yin D, Gery S, Kawamata N, Takai N, Komatsu, N, Chumakov, A, Imai Y, Koeffler HP (2007) Histone deacetylase inhibitor, suberoylanilide hydroxamic acid (Vorinostat, SAHA) profoundly inhibits the growth of human pancreatic cancer cells. *Int J Cancer* 121:656-665.

Lagger GO, Carroll D, Rembold M, Khier H, Tischler J, Weitzer G, huettengruber B, Hauser C, Brunmeir R, Jenuwein T, Seiser C (2002) Essential function of histone deacetylase 1 in proliferation control and CDK inhibitor repression. *EMBO J* 21:2672-2681.

Lakshmikanthan V, Kaddour-Djebbar I, Lewis RW, Kumar MV (2006) SAHA-sensitized prostate cancer cells to TNF alpha-related apoptosis-inducing ligand (TRAIL): mechanisms leading to synergistic apoptosis. *Int J Cancer* 119:221-228.

Larsen L, Tonnesen M, Ronn SG, Størling J, Jørgensen S, Mascagni P, Dinarello CA, Billestrup N, Mandrup-Poulsen T (2007) Inhibition of histone deacetylases prevents cytokine-induced toxicity in beta cells. *Diabetologia* 50:779-789.

Lathia, JD, Mack SC, Mulkearns-Hubert EE, Valentim CL, Rich JN (2015) Cancer stem cells in glioblastoma. *Genes Dev* 29:1203-1217.

Levine B, Kroemer G (2008) Autophagy in the pathogenesis of disease. *Cell* 132:27-42.

Li Y, Dai D, Lu Q, Fei M, Li M and Wu, x (2013) Sirt2 suppresses glioma cell growth through targeting NF-κB-miR-21 axis. *Biochem Biophys Res Commun* 441:661-667.

Li Y, Seto E (2016) HDACs and HDAC Inhibitors in cancer development and therapy. *Cold Spring Harb Perspect Med* 6:1-34.

Liby P, Kostrouchova M, Pohludka M, Yilma P, Hrabal P, Sikora J, Brožova E, Kostrouchova M Rall JE, Kostrouch Z (2006) Elevated and deregulated expression of HDAC3 in human astrocytic glial tumours. *Folia Biol (Praha)* 52:21-33.

Licciardi PV, Karagiannis TC (2012) Regulation of immune responses by histone deacetylase inhibitors. *ISRN Hematol* 2012:690901.

Lin HY, Chen CS, Lin SP, Weng JR, Chen CS (2006) Targeting histone deacetylase in cancer therapy. *Med Res Rev* 26:397-413.

Liu H, Hu Q, Kaufman A, Joseph D'Ercole A, Ye P (2008) Developmental expression of histone deacetylase 11 in the murine brain. *J Neurosci Res* 86:537-543.

Liu T, Liu PY, Marshall GM (2009) The critical role of the class III histone deacetylase SIRT1 in cancer. *Cancer Res* 69:1702-1705.

Liu T, Tee AE, Porro A, Smith SA, Dwarte T, Liu PY, Iraci N, Sekyere E, Haber M, Norris MD, Diolaiti G, Della Valle G, Perini G, Marshall GM (2007) Activation of tissue transglutaminase transcription by histone deacetylase inhibition as a therapeutic approach for Myc oncogenesis. *Proc Natl Acad Sci USA* 104:18682-18687.

Liu YL, Yang PM, Shun CT, Wu MS, Weng JR, Chen CC (2010) Autophagy potentiates the anti-cancer effects of the histone deacetylase inhibitors in hepatocellular carcinoma. *Autophagy* 6:1057-1065.

Loffet A, (2002) Peptides as drugs: is there a market? *J Pept Sci* 8:1-7.

Lucio-Eterovic AK, Cortez MA, Valera ET, Motta FJ, Queiroz RG, Machado HR, Carlotti CG, Neder L, Scrideli CA, Tone LG (2008)

Differential expression of 12 histone deacetylase (HDAC) genes in astrocytomas and normal brain tissue: class II and IV are hypoexpressed in glioblastomas. *BMC Cancer* 8:243.

MacDonald JL, Roskams AJ (2008) Histone deacetylases 1 and 2 are expressed at distinct stages of neuro-glial development. *Dev Dyn* 237:2256–2267.

Macenka DG, Olivi A (2011) Patients' Guide to Brain Cancer. In: *Johns Hopkins Medicine* (Shockney LD, Shapiro GR, editors) Jones & Bartlett Learning, Sudbury, MA, USA.

Mann SB, Johnson JR, Cohen MH, Justice R, Pazdur R (2007) FDA approval summary: Vorinostat for treatment of advanced primary cutaneous T-cell lymphoma. *The Oncologist*. 12:1247-1252.

Marks PA (2007) Discovery and development of SAHA as an anticancer agent. *Oncogene* 26:1351-1356.

Marks PA (2010) Histone deacetylase inhibitors: a chemical genetics approach to understanding cellular functions. *Biochim Biophys Acta* 1799:717-725.

Marks PA and Breslow R (2007) Dimethyl sulfoxide to Vorinostat: development of this histone deacetylase inhibitor as an anticancer drug. *Nat Biotechnol* 25:84-90.

Marks PA, Rifkind RA, Richon VM, Breslow R, Miller T, Kelly WK (2001) Histone deacetylases and cancer: causes and therapies. *Nat Rev Cancer* 1:194-202.

Marks PA, Sheffery M, Rifkind RA (1987) Induction of transformed cells to terminal differentiation and the modulation of gene expression. *Cancer Res* 47:659-666.

Mathew R, Karp CM, Beaudoin B, Vuong N, Chen G, Chen, HY (2009) Autophagy suppresses tumorigenesis through elimination of p62. *Cell* 137:1062-1075.

Mazure NM, Pouyssegur J (2010) Hypoxia-induced autophagy: cell death or cell survival. *Curr Opin Cell Biol* 22:177-180.

Miller TA, Witter DJ, Belvedere S (2003) Histone deacetylase inhibitors. *J Med Chem* 46:5097-5116.

Mohan N, Banik NL, Ray SK (2011) Synergistic efficacy of a novel combination therapy controls growth of Bcl-x_L bountiful neuroblastoma cells by increasing differentiation and apoptosis. *Cancer Biol Ther* 12:846-854.

Mohan N, Chakrabarti M, Banik NL, Ray SK (2013) Combination of LC3 shRNA plasmid transfection and genistein treatment inhibited autophagy and increased apoptosis in malignant neuroblastoma in cell culture and animal models. *PLoS One* 8:e78958.

Mottamal M, Zheng S, Huang TL, Wang G (2015) Histone deacetylase inhibitors in clinical studies as templates for new anticancer agents. *Molecules* 20:3898-3941.

Munster PN, Troso-Sandoval T, Rosen N, Rifkind R, Marks PA, Richon VM (2001) The histone deacetylase inhibitor suberoylanilide hydroxamic acid induces differentiation of human breast cancer. *Cancer Res* 61:8492-8497.

Namdar M, Perez G, Ngo L, Marks PM (2010) Selective inhibition of histone deacetylase 6 (HDAC6) induces DNA damage and sensitizes transformed cells to anticancer agents. *Proc Natl Acad USA* 107:20003-20008.

Nishida K, Komiyama T, Miyazawa S, Shen ZN, Furumatsu T, Doi H, Yoshida A, Yamana J, Yamamura M, Ninomiya Y, Inoue H, Asahara H (2004) Histone deacetylase inhibitor suppression of autoantibody-mediated arthritis in mice via regulation of p16INK4a and p21(WAF1/Cip1) expression. *Arthritis Rheum* 50:3365-3376.

Orzan F, Pellegatta S, Poliani PL, Pisati F, Caldera V, Menghi F, Kapetis D, Marras C, Schiffer D, Finocchiaro, G (2011) Enhancer of Zeste 2 (EZH2) is up-regulated in malignant gliomas and in glioma stem-like cells. *Neuropathol Appl Neurobiol* 37:381-394.

Ostrom QT, Gittleman H, Fulop J, Liu M, Blanda R, Kromer C, Wolinsky Y, Kruchko C, Barnholtz-Sloan JS (2015) CBTRUS Statistical report: primary brain and central nervous system tumors diagnosed in the United States in 2008-2012. *Neuro Oncol* 17:iv1-iv62.

Ostrom QT, Gittleman H, Fulop J, Liu M, Blanda RC, Wolinsky Y, Kruchko C, Barnholtz-Sloan JS (2016) CBTRUS Statistical report:

primary brain and central nervous system tumors diagnosed in the United States in 2009-2013. *Neuro Oncol* 18:v1-v75.

Papi A, Ferreri AM, Rocchi P, Guerra F, Orlandi M (2010) Epigenetic modifiers as anticancer drugs: effectiveness of valproic acid in neural crest-derived tumor cells. *Anticancer Res* 30:535-540.

Park JH, Kim SH, Choi MC, Lee J, Oh DY, Im SA, Bang YJ, Kim TY (2008) Class II histone deacetylases play pivotal roles in heat shock protein 90-mediated proteasomal degradation of vascular endothelial growth factor receptors. *Biochem Biophys Res Commun* 368:318-322.

Peart MJ, Smyth GK, Van Laar RK, Bowtell DD, Richon VM, Marks PA, Holloway AJ, Johnstone RW (2005) Identification and functional significance of genes regulated by structurally different histone deacetylase inhibitors. *Proc Natl Acad Sci USA* 102:16090-16095.

Qu Y, Zhang J, Wu S, Li B, Liu S, Cheng J (2012) SIRT1 promotes proliferation and inhibits apoptosis of human malignant glioma cell lines. *Neurosci Lett* 525:168-172.

Rasmussen RD, Gajjar MK, Jensen KE, Hamerlik P (2016) Enhanced efficacy of combined HDAC and PARP targeting in glioblastoma. *Mol Oncol* 10:751-763.

Ray SK (2016) The transcription regulator Krüppel-like factor 4 and its dual roles of oncogene in glioblastoma and tumor suppressor in neuroblastoma. *For Immunopathol Dis Therap* 7:127-139.

Rettig I, Koeneke E, Trippel F, Mueller WC, Burhenne J, Kopp-Schneider A, Fabian J, Schober A, Fernekorn U, Von Deimling A, Deubzer HE, Milde T, Witt O, Oehme I (2015) Selective inhibition of HDAC8 decreases neuroblastoma growth in vitro and in vivo and enhances retinoic acid-mediated differentiation. *Cell Death Dis* 6:e1657.

Richon VM (2006) Cancer biology: mechanism of antitumour action of vorinostat (suberoylanilide hydroxamic acid), a novel histone deacetylase inhibitor. *Br J Cancer* 95:S2-S6.

Richon VM, Webb Y, Merger R, Sheppard T, Jursic B, Ngo L, Civoli F, Breslow R, Rifflikn RA, Mark PM (1996) Second generation hybrid polar compounds are potent inducers of transformed cell differentiation. *Proc Natl Acad Sci USA* 93:5705-5708.

Rikiishi H (2011) Autophagic and apoptotic effects of HDAC inhibitors on cancer cells. *J Biomed Biotechnol* 2011:830260.

Robert T, Vanoli F, Chiolo I, Shubassi G, Bernstein KA, Rothstein R, Foiani M (2011). HDACs link the DNA damage response, processing of double-strand breaks and autophagy. *Nature* 471:74-79.

Ropero S, Esteller M (2007) The role of histone deacetylases (HDACs) in human cancer. *Mol Oncol* 1:19-25.

Rosato RR, Almenara JA, Grant S (2003) The histone deacetylase inhibitor MS-275 promotes differentiation or apoptosis in human leukemia cells through a process regulated by generation of reactive oxygen species and induction of p21Cip1/Waf1. *Cancer Res* 63:3637-3645.

Roy Choudhury S, Karmakar S, Banik NL, Ray SK (2011) Valproic acid induced differentiation and potentiated efficacy of taxol and nanotaxol for controlling growth of human glioblastoma LN18 and T98G cells. *Neurochem Res* 36:2292-2305.

Sarcar B, Kahali B, Chinnaiyan P (2010) Vorinostat enhances the cytotoxic effects of the topoisomerase I inhibitor SN38 in glioblastoma cell lines. *J Neuro-Oncol* 99:201- 207.

Sawa H, Murakami H, Kumagai M, Nakasato M, Yamauchi S, Matsuyama Yasuo N, Akira Satone T, Ikuo Hashimoto W, Kamada H (2004) Histone deacetylase inhibitor, FK228, induces apoptosis and suppresses cell proliferation of human glioblastoma cells in vitro and in vivo. *Acta Neuropathol* 107:523-531.

Schmoch T, Gal Z, Mock A, Mossemann J, Lahrmann B, Grabe N, Schmezer P, Lasitschka F, Beckhove P, Unterberg A, Herold-Mende C (2016) Combined treatment of ATRA with epigenetic drugs increases aggressiveness of glioma xenografts. *Anticancer Res* 36:1489-1496.

Shabason JE, Tofilon PJ, Camphausen K (2011) Grand rounds at the National Institutes of Health: HDAC inhibitors as radiation modifiers, from bench to clinic. *J Cell Mol Med* 12:2735-2744.

Sikandar S, Dizon D, Shen X, Li Z, Besterman J, Lipkin SM (2010) The class I HDAC inhibitor MGCD0103 induces cell cycle arrest and apoptosis in colon cancer initiating cells by upregulating Dickkopf-1 and non-canonical Wnt signaling. *Oncotarget* 1:596-605.

Silva G, Cardoso BA, Belo H, Almeida AM (2013) Vorinostat induces apoptosis and differentiation in myeloid malignancies: genetic and molecular mechanisms. *PLoS One* 8:e53766.

Singh BN, Zhang G, Hwa YL, Li G, Dowdy SC, Jiang S (2010) Non-histone protein acetylation as cancer therapy targets. *Expert Rev Anticancer Ther* 6:935–954.

Singh MM, Johnson B, Venkatarayan A, Flores ER, Zhang J, Su X, Barton M Lang F, Chandra J (2015) Preclinical activity of combined HDAC and KDM1A inhibition in glioblastoma. *Neuro Oncol* 17:1463-1473.

Skov S, Rieneck K, Bovin LF, Skak K, Tomra S, Michelsen BK, Ødum, N (2003) Histone deacetylase inhibitors: a new class of immunosuppressors targeting a novel signal pathway essential for CD154 expression. *Blood* 101:1430-1438.

Spalletta G, Cravello L, Piras F, Iorio M, Sancesario G, Marchi A, Caltagirone C, Cacciari C (2013) Rapid-onset apathy may be the only clinical manifestation after dorsal striatum hemorrhagic lesion: a case report. *Alzheimer Dis Assoc Disord* 27:192-194.

Struhl K (1998) Histone acetylation and transcriptional regulatory mechanisms. *Genes Dev* 12:599-606.

Sugo N, Oshiro H, Takemura M, Kobayashi T, Kohno Y, Uesaka N, Song WJ, Yamamoto N (2010) Nucleocytoplasmic translocation of HDAC9 regulates gene expression and dendritic growth in developing cortical neurons. *Eur J Neurosci* 31:1521-1532.

Sun GQ, Yu RT, Evans RM, Shi Y (2007) Orphan nuclear receptor TLX recruits histone deacetylases to repress transcription and regulate neural stem cell proliferation. *Proc Natl Acad Sci USA* 104:15282-15287.

Suzuki K, Ohsumi Y (2007) Molecular machinery of autophagosome formation in yeast, *Saccharomyces cerevisiae*. *FEBS Lett* 581:2156-2161.

Svechnikova I, Almqvist PM, Ekström, TJ (2008) HDAC inhibitors effectively induce cell type-specific differentiation in human glioblastoma cell lines of different origin. *Int J Oncol* 32:821-827.

Takahashi N (2002) Induction of cell differentiation and development of new anticancer drugs. *Yakugaku Zasshi* 122:547-563.

Tang D, Kang R, Livesey KM, Cheh CW, Farkas A, Loughran P, Hoppe G, Bianchi ME, Tracey KJ, Zeh HJ, Lotze MT (2010) Endogenous HMGB1 regulates autophagy. *J Cell Biol* 190:881-892.

Townsend PA, Crabb SJ, Davidson SM, Johnson PWM, Packham G, Ganesan A (2007) The bicyclic depsipeptide family of histone deacetylase inhibitors. In: *Chemical Biology from Small Molecules to System Biology and Drug Design* (Schreiber SL, Kapoor TM, Wess G, editors), Vol. 1-3, Wiley-VCH, Weinheim, Germany, p.693-720.

Tseng, JH, Chen, CY, Chen, PC, Hsiao, SH, Fan, CC, Liang, YC and Chen, CP (2017) Valproic acid inhibits glioblastoma multiforme cell growth via paraoxonase 2 expression. *Oncotarget* 8:14666-14679.

Ueda H, Nakajima H, Hori Y, Fujita T, Nishimura M, Goto T, Okuhara M. (1994) Action of FR901228, a novel antitumor bicyclic depsipeptide produced by *Chromobacterium violaceum* No. 968, on Ha-ras transformed NIH3T3 cells. *Biosci Biotechnol Biochem* 58:1579-1583.

Ugur HC, Ramakrishna N, Bello L, Menon LG, Kim SK, Black PM, Carroll RS (2007) Continuous intracranial administration of suberoylanilide hydroxamic acid (SAHA) inhibits tumor growth in an orthotopic glioma model. *J Neuro-oncol* 83:267-275.

Valk-Lingbeek ME, Bruggeman SW, van Lohuizen M (2004) Stem cells and cancer; the Polycomb connection. *Cell* 118:409-418.

Wade, PA (2001) Transcriptional control at regulatory checkpoints by histone deacetylases: molecular connections between cancer and chromatin. *Hum Mol Genet* 10:693-698.

Wallace GC 4th, Haar CP, Vandergrift WA 3rd, Giglio P, Dixon-Mah YN, Varma AK, Ray SK, Patel SJ, Banik NL, Das A (2013) Multi-targeted DATS prevents tumor progression and promotes apoptosis in ectopic glioblastoma xenografts in SCID mice via HDAC inhibition. *J Neuro oncol* 114:43-50.

Wang AH, Betos NR, Vezmar M, Pelletier N, Crosato M, Heng HH, Th'ng J, Han J, Yang XJ (1999) HDAC4, a human histone deacetylase related to yeast HDAC1, is a transcriptional corepressor. *Mol Cell Biol* 19:7816-7827.

Wang YC, Yang X, Xing LH, Kong WZ (2013) Effects of SAHA on proliferation and apoptosis of hepatocellular carcinoma cells and hepatitis B virus replication. *World J Gastroenterol* 19:5159-5164.

Wang Z, Hu P, Tang F, Lian H, Chen X, Zhang Y, He X, Liu W, Xie C (2016) HDAC6 promotes cell proliferation and confers resistance to temozolomide in glioblastoma. *Cancer Lett* 379:134-42.

Wei L, Hong S, Yoon Y, Hwang SN, Park JC, Zhang Z, Olson JJ, Hu XP, Shim H (2012) Early prediction of response to Vorinostat in an orthotopic rat glioma model. *NMR Biomed* 25:1104-1111.

Weichert W (2009) HDAC expression and clinical prognosis in human malignancies. *Cancer Lett* 280:168-176.

White E (2012) Deconvoluting the context-dependent role for autophagy in cancer. *Nat Rev Cancer* 12:401-410.

White E (2016) Autophagy and p53. *Cold Spring Harb Perspect Med* 6:a026120.

Wilson AJ, Byun DS, Popova N, Murray LB, L'Italien K, Sowa Y, Arango D, Velcich A, Augenlicht LH, Mariadason JM. (2006). Histone deacetylase 3 (HDAC3) and other class I HDACs regulate colon cell maturation and p21 expression and are deregulated in human colon cancer. *J Biol Chem* 281:13548-13558.

Wolf IM, Fan Z, Rauh M, Seufert S, Hore N, Buchfelder M, Savaskan NE, Eyüpoglu IY (2014) Histone deacetylases inhibition by SAHA/Vorinostat normalizes the glioma microenvironment via xCT equilibration. *Sci Rep* 4:6226.

Wu Z, Jing S, Li Y, Gao Y, Yu S, Li Z, Zhao Y, Piao J, Ma S, Chen X (2017) The effects of SAHA on radiosensitivity in pancreatic cancer cells by inducing apoptosis and targeting RAD51. *Biomed Pharmacother* 89:705-710.

Yang ZJ, Chee CE, Huang S, Sinicrope FA (2011) The role of autophagy in cancer: therapeutic implications. *Mol Cancer Ther* 10:1533-1541.

Yin D, Ong JM, Hu J, Desmond JC, Kawamata N, Konda BM, Black KL, Koeffler HP (2007) Suberoylanilide hydroxamic acid, a histone deacetylase inhibitor: effects on gene expression and growth of glioma cells in vitro and in vivo. *Clin Cancer Res* 13:1045-1052.

Yoshida M, Matsuyama A, Komatsu A, Nishino N (2003) From discovery to the coming generation of histone deacetylase inhibitors. *Curr Med Chem* 10:2351-2358.

Zhang R, Banik NL, Ray SK (2008) Combination of all-*trans* retinoic acid and interferon-gamma upregulated p27(Kip1) and down regulated CDK2 to cause cell cycle arrest leading to differentiation and apoptosis in human glioblastoma LN18 (PTEN-proficient) and U87MG (PTEN-deficient) cells. *Cancer Chemother Pharmacol* 62:407-416.

Zhang X, Han S, Kang Y, Guo M, Hong S, Liu F, Fu S, Wang L, Wang Q (2012) SAHA, an HDAC inhibitor, synergizes with tacrolimus to prevent murine cardiac allograft rejection. *Cell Mol Immunol* 9:390-398.

Zhang, XD, Gillespie, SK, Borrow, JM, Hersey, P (2004) The histone deacetylase inhibitor suberic bishydroxamate regulates the expression of multiple apoptotic mediators and induces mitochondria-dependent apoptosis of melanoma cells. *Mol Cancer Ther* 3:425-435.

Zhao Y, Tan J, Zhuang L, Jiang X, Liu ET, Yu Q (2005) Inhibitors of histone deacetylases target the Rb-E2F1 pathway for apoptosis induction through activation. *Proc Natl Acad Sci USA* 102:16090-16095.

In: Horizons in Neuroscience Research ISBN: 978-1-53613-286-1
Editors: A. Costa and E. Villalba

Chapter 2

MOTION-INDUCED BLINDNESS AND THE SPINNING DANCER PARADIGM: A NEURONAL NETWORK APPROACH BASED ON SYNERGETICS

T. D. Frank [*] ***and J. O'Leary***
Department of Psychology, University of Connecticut, Storrs, CT, US

ABSTRACT

Motion-induced blindness occurs when a stationary foreground pattern is not or only partially perceived due to a moving background pattern although it is not obscured by the moving background pattern. Periods of blindness alternate with periods of clear perception. Perception is oscillatory. Likewise, the so-called spinning dancer movie presenting a silhouetted rotating dancer figure induces oscillatory perception. Periods in which the dancer is perceived to rotate clockwise alternate with periods in which the dancer is perceived to rotate counter-clockwise although during both periods the movie plays the same frames. Two experiments are reported to illustrate the motion-induced blindness and spinning

[*] Corresponding Author Email: till.frank@uconn.edu.

dancer paradigms. Subsequently, a neuronal network approach is presented to explain the oscillatory perceptual dynamics. The neuronal network approach is based on synergetics, a theory of pattern formation and self-organization. Accordingly, the theoretical framework explains perceptual oscillations in terms of a self-regulated alternation of brain activity patterns.

Keywords: perceptual ambiguity, perceptual oscillations, neuronal networks, synergetics

INTRODUCTION

The self-organization perspective of human perception and behavior provides a general theoretical framework to address various aspects of human perception and behavior from a unified point of view (Haken, 1996; Kelso, 1995). In particular, observed brain activity patterns as measured by encephalography (Haken, 1996; Kelso, 1995) as well as neuronal network modeling (Haken, 1991) can be taken into consideration when discussing how individuals perceive objects and perform certain behaviors. Importantly, just as any theoretical framework, the self-organization perspective as a theoretical framework comes with certain interpretations of experimental observations that might motivate further experimental efforts. In this chapter, perceptual oscillations induced by seemingly ambiguous or conflicting dynamic circumstances of the visual world will be addressed from the aforementioned self-organization perspective. The oscillatory nature of perceptual oscillations will be interpreted as an interplay between two processes: self-organization processes, on the one hand, and processes of neuronal network restructuration reflecting neuronal plasticity, on the other hand. Let us turn first to the phenomenon of perceptual oscillations.

Objects in the world of an individual are composed of atoms and molecules and exhibit various properties such as shape and color. Nevertheless, a given object at a particular point of time can be described by individuals in different ways. Individuals may refer to a glass filled halfway with water as a glass that is half full or as a glass that is half empty. A benchmark example of a stationary figure that allows for two interpretations is the Necker cube (Attneave, 1971; Brosellino et al., 1972). The cube might be interpreted as an object that points down to the left or as an object that points upwards to the right. Observers viewing a Necker cube perceive one of the two interpretations for a particular period. Subsequently, the perception switches and the alternative interpretation is perceived for a certain period. After that, the perception of the Necker cube switches again and so on. As a result, perception of the Necker cube is an oscillatory process. Frequently, the human brain is considered as a computer and it is assumed that the human brain would compute or process something (Goldstein, 2010; Mamassian and Landy, 1998; Mamassian and Goutcher, 2005). In particular, it is assumed the brain would process information. Accordingly, it is assumed that there would be ambiguous circumstances of the visual world that do not contain sufficient information such that computational processes cannot yield unique solutions (Mamassian et al., 1998, 2005).

While the Necker cube and similar figures (Haken, 1991) are stationary figures, there are dynamic (i.e., nonstationary) conditions of the visual world that are seemingly ambiguous. The spinning dancer movie is a benchmark example in this regard. The video shows a female three-dimensional silhouetted dancer in black rotating in front of a gray background. In this context, the question arises in which direction does the dancer rotate: clockwise or counterclockwise? In fact, observers report that the figure rotates in one direction (e.g., clockwise) for a period and then suddenly switches the rotation direction and rotates in the opposite direction (e.g., counter-clockwise). Then rotation direction switches again and again. In summary, the perception of the rotation direction switches in an oscillatory fashion. Note that here and above, the phrase oscillatory is used. In fact, the phenomenon features an alternation between two states just like if someone is switching a light on and off repeatedly. Nevertheless, in what follows the phrase oscillatory will be used because it is assumed that the underlying brain activity changes in an oscillatory fashion like a pendulum (see below). These discrete and continuous pictures of the same issue are not inconsistent with each other. The reader may think of a swinging pendulum that swings from left to right. Then, let us assume that there is an observer who switches a light on and off every time when the pendulum assumes its most left or most right position, respectively. Then the continuous oscillations of the pendulum produce an alternating temporal pattern between two discrete states (the on and off states). Liu et al. (2012) tested participants under the spinning dancer paradigm. They found that when participants focused on the feet of the dancer the rotation direction switched more frequently as compared to an experimental condition in which participants focused on the body of the dancer. Moreover, consistent with earlier work on the Necker cube perception (Kornmeier et al., 2009), Liu et al. (2012) found that the cognitive state of the individual as manipulated by appropriate instructions can affect the frequency of the experienced switches.

Various studies have determined characteristic features of brain activity during perceptual oscillations. For the Necker cube paradigm, brain activity before and after perceptual switching events has been compared to brain activity during periods in which observers did not experience perceptual switching (Britz et al., 2009, Kornmeier and Bach, 2004). For another stationary experimental design based on perceptual rivalry similar findings have been obtained (Leopold and Logothetis, 1999; Sterzer et al., 2009). For a seemingly ambiguous visual world scenario based on apparent motion that leads to oscillatory perception, features of brain activity have been identified that are characteristic for perceptual switches to occur (Mueller et al., 1999, 2005). In contrast to the aforementioned studies on the Necker cube and rivalry paradigm, which involve stationary external circumstances, apparent motion experiments involve objects (e.g., dots) that seem to move. Consequently, apparent motion experiments are about dynamic external circumstances just like experiments utilizing the spinning dancer movie or other movies.

Motion-induced blindness (MIB) is a figure-ground perception phenomenon in which the background rotates, while the foreground is stationary. In a typical MIB experiment, a field of dots is rotating in the background, while a small number of dots with different color are stationary in the foreground. Observers viewing the foreground pattern experience that parts of the foreground pattern disappear for certain periods of time. In this sense, observers become blind to details of the foreground figures presented to them. The MIB phenomena has been examined under various conditions (Bonneh et al., 2001). In particular, it has been shown that the number of disappearances per time increases when the rotation speed of the background pattern increases. Moreover, it has been shown that rate of MIB disappearances (the number of disappearances per time) is positively correlated with the rate of switches in a perceptual rivalry experiment (Carter and Pettigrew, 2003). Perceptual rivalry, in turn, has been suggested to arise due to competitive interaction between activity of the left and right hemispheres of the human brain (Pettigrew, 2001).

The MIB phenomenon just as the spinning dancer perception is considered an oscillatory perceptual phenomenon. Periods in which the foreground pattern is clearly perceived alternate with periods in which the whole or parts of the foreground pattern disappear.

Although it has been acknowledged (Pettigrew, 2001) that perceptual oscillations as reported above are likely caused by bistable brain oscillators (in the sense of the aforementioned continuously oscillating pendulum that produces discrete on and off states), little effort has been directed to address such a bistable brain oscillator from a self-organization perspective. In what follows, we will report from two experiments of oscillatory perception using spinning dancer and MIB paradigms. Subsequently, following earlier work of Ditzinger and Haken (1989) and others (Frank, 2014, 2015; Haken 1991), oscillatory perception will be modeled on the basis of a neuronal network model that describes alternating phases of self-organization and neuronal network restructuring. Finally, our experimental results and previously published results will be discussed with respect to the proposed model.

METHODS

Participants

Thirteen University of Connecticut undergraduate students participated. Data from one participant were discarded because the participant in one condition did not exhibit perceptual oscillations at all. The age of the remaining twelve participants (7 female, 5 male) was M = 19 year (SD = 1). All participants were right handed. All participants had normal or corrected to normal vision. Subjects received course credits for their participation.

Materials

For Experiment 1, the spinning dancer video designed by Nobuyuki Kayahara (available at http://www.procreo.jp/labo/labo13) was used. The video showed a three-dimensional silhouetted female dancer in black which rotated continuously in front of a gray background. The video was displayed on a computer screen. For Experiment 2, a motion-induced blindness video was used designed by Michael Bach (available at www.michaelbach.de/ot/mot-mib). The video showed a squared grid composed of 7 times 7 crosses in blue color that rotated clockwise in front of a black background with adjustable rotation speed. In the foreground the video showed three yellow dots that were stationary. Dot size was fixed to 3 units. The background was black. The video was displayed on the same screen as the spinning dancer video. Each video was presented separately.

Design and Analysis

In Experiment 1 (spinning dancer experiment), there was one dependent variable, which was the frequency (or number) of the perceived switches of the dancer from clockwise to counter clockwise spinning and vice versa. There were two independent variables. The first independent variable was focus. Participants were told to focus on either the top (body) of the dancer or the bottom (feet). The second factor was the block number. The two levels of the first independent variables were administered in a first and a second block such that each focus condition was repeated twice. In Experiment 2 (MIB experiment) the dependent variable was the number of disappearances of the yellow dots in the reporting period. The independent variable was the speed in rotations per minutes (RPM) and had 3 levels (1, 11, and 21 RPM). The 3 levels were presented in a sequence. Each participant was test twice with a 3-speed sequence. Scores were averaged across the two sequences (i.e., the factor block was ignored). Experiments 1 and 2 were counterbalanced such that some participants were tested in Experiment 1 first and in Experiment 2 second, whereas other participants were tested in Experiment 2 first and in Experiment 1 second. Within Experiments 1 and 2 conditions were counterbalanced as well.

Procedure

For both experiments, participants were seated one meter away from the computer screen. For Experiment 1 (spinning dancer) the procedure was as follows. Depending on the focus condition, participants were told to focus on the body or feet of the dancer. Participants were instructed to inform the experimenter when they saw the dancer switching the spinning direction. They were told to say "now" out loud when a switch happened. They watched the spinning dancer video in a given focus condition for 3 minutes. Between conditions short breaks of less than a minute were allowed. Consequently, the whole experiment took between 12 and 15 minutes. For Experiment 2 (MIB experiment) the procedure was as follows. Participants watched the MIB video in a sequence with three different rotation speeds (1, 11, and 21 RPM). Each speed condition was presented for 1 minute. Between speed conditions there were no breaks.

The speed conditions were either presented in ascending (1, 11, and 21 RPM) or descending (21, 11, 1 RPM) order. Each participant was test only on one type of presentation order. The order was counterbalanced across participants. The 3-speed sequences were presented twice. Between these two blocks there was a 1 minute break. Just as in Experiment 1, in Experiment 2 participants were instructed to say "now" out loud every time they experienced a disappearance whether it was the disappearance of one, two or all three target dots. At the end of Experiments 1 and 2 participants were debriefed about the nature of the two experiments. That is, they were informed that the switches were illusions and that the computer was not creating the switches.

RESULTS

First, the results of the spinning dancer experiment will be presented. Figure 1 shows the number of switches between clockwise and counterclockwise rotations of the spinning dancer for the two focus conditions and two repetitions. In both blocks, participants experienced more switches when they focused on the lower part of the spinning dancer. Consequently, when averaging scores across blocks, we found that scores were higher in the lower part focus condition (M = 10.8, SD = 6.9) as compared to the upper part focus condition (M = 8.9, SD = 5.0). Moreover, as can be seen from Figure 1, overall, the number of switches increased from block 1 (M = 8.8, SD = 5.0) to block 2 (M = 11.0, SD = 6.1). A 2x2 ANOVA showed that the main effect of block was statistically significant, $F(1, 11) = 6.724$, $p < 0.05$. In contrast, the main effect of focus and the interaction effect were not statistically significant.

Let us present next the results from the MIB experiment. For 1 RPM on the average M = 4.3 (SD = 4.8) disappearances were observed. For 11 RPM on the average M = 21.2 (SD = 8.8) disappearances were observed. Finally, for 21 RPM on the average M = 28.1 (SD = 14.0) disappearances were observed. The number of disappearances increased as a function of rotation speed. One-way ANOVA showed that the effect of speed was statistically significant, $F(2, 22) = 29.030$, $p < 0.001$. Trend analysis showed that the linear trend was statistically significant, $F(1, 11) = 32.883$, $p < 0.001$.

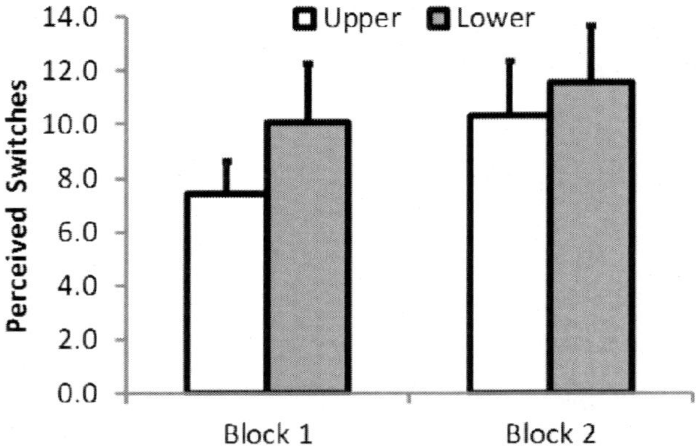

Figure 1. Perceived switches as function of focus and block. Error bars represent standard errors of means.

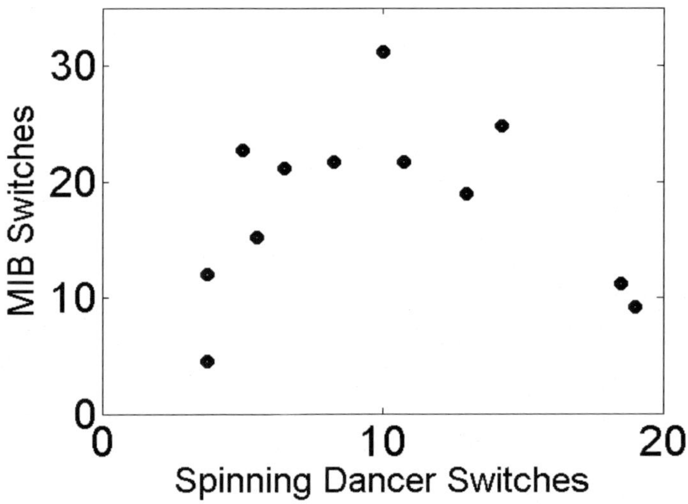

Figure 2. Scatter plot illustrating the correlation between performance measures of Experiments 1 and 2. Number of disappearances (switches between complete and incomplete perceptions) observed in the motion-induced blindness (MIB) experiment are plotted versus the number of switches in rotation direction observed in the spinning dancer experiment.

Finally, Figure 2 shows the scatter plot of the overall performance scores from Experiments 1 (spinning dancer) and 2 (MIB). The scores formed an inverted U shaped pattern.

Discussion of Experimental Results

In Experiment 1, it was found that the number of switches during the observation period was higher when participants focused on the feet of the dancer as compared to the condition in which participants focused on the body of the dancer. This effect of focus is consistent with the study by Liu et al. (2012). However, while in the study by Liu et al. (2012) the difference between the focus condition reached statistical significant, in our study, it did not. The reason for this might be that Liu et al. (2012) used a larger sample size (about 20 participants) and longer viewing times (about 20 minutes). Liu et al. (2012) did not consider time as a factor. In contrast, we distinguished between two time blocks. We found that the number of switches increased over time slightly. This effect of time reached statistical significance. It is known from other perceptual oscillation phenomena that the oscillation rate (or the switching rate) increases initially and eventually reaches a saturation value (e.g., in experiments on the Necker cube viewing, see Haken, 1991). Therefore, block 1 is considered to be a transient phase reflecting neuronal plasticity of the perceptual system on a times scale of minutes.

In Experiment 2, we found that the number of disappearances increased as a function of the rotation speed of the background pattern. Although the variability in terms of standard deviations was relatively large with respect to the mean values, a detailed look at the individual data revealed that the scores increased from the 1 RPM to the 11 RPM condition for all participants. From the 11 RPM to the 21 RPM condition, the scores increased for 10 out of 12 participants and decreased for the remaining 2. Therefore, the effect of speed had a robust effect on the participants irrespective of their individual (and different) overall performance scores. The observed effect of speed on the number of disappearances was previously reported by Bonneh et al. (2001).

Since our participants performed in both experiments, we were able to produce a scatter plot of the number of MIB disappearances versus the number of spinning dancer switches, see Figure 2. The scatter plot reveals a nonlinear pattern in the form of an inverted U. A possible interpretation of the inverted U pattern is that our participants represented two different populations with correlations in opposing directions. Accordingly, the participants with relative few spinning dancer switches (below 10) would exhibit a positive linear correlation, while the participants with a relative large number of spinning dancer switches (above 10) would exhibit a negative linear correlation. The overlapping of these two linear patterns of correlations would yield the observed scatter plot. Support for this speculation may be found in studies that have identified linear correlations between different types of perceptual oscillations. Carter and Pettigrew (2003) found a positive correlation between rate of MIB disappearances and the switching rate observed in a perceptual rivalry experiment. Sheppard and Pettigrew (2006) found a positive correlation between the switching rate observed in the same kind of perceptual rivalry experiment and the rate of perceptual oscillations induced by a moving plaid pattern. Having said that, while in both aforementioned studies (Carter et al., 2003; Sheppard et al., 2006) positive correlation have been identified, the inverted U shaped pattern hints that negative correlations might occur as well at least in certain sub-populations of the general population.

SELF-ORGANIZATION PERSPECTIVE AND MODELLING

From a self-organization perspective brain activity patterns related to percepts (or perceptual experiences) are self-organized patterns. They emerge due to bifurcations. The external circumstances as manipulated in experiments (in particular the experiments reported above) in general have two impacts: they set the initial conditions for the formation of the patterns and affect the neuronal network structure and the general structure (e.g., posture-related structure) of an individual under consideration. Although the self-organization, pattern formation perspective allows for neuronal network modeling, the perspective differs from classical neuronal network approaches that are based on notions such as information processing and computation.

According to the self-organization perspective, seemingly ambiguous situations arise from symmetry properties of the human self-organizing system. Figure 3 illustrates this point. Let us consider panel A first. Let us consider a chemical reaction in a container with a square boundary. The reaction is assumed to exhibit a bifurcation point that is defined by certain critical concentrations of the substances involved in the reaction. Below that bifurcation point the concentrations of all substances are constant across space such that the system exhibits no pattern (or a spatially homogeneous pattern). In contrast, it is assumed that slightly above the bifurcation point a stripe pattern with a well-defined period emerges. The stripe pattern is oriented parallel to the boundaries of the container. From the geometry of the container it follows that two stripe patterns can emerge: one pattern orientated in the X direction, the other in the Y direction. Let us assume that these two patterns are competitive. Then only one pattern can emerge at a time. In summary, when the chemical system is prepared slightly above its bifurcation point it exhibits two possible patterns and in this sense is in a seemingly ambiguous condition. The seemingly ambiguity arises from the symmetry of the self-organizing system. The ambiguity is only an apparent ambiguity. For any initial condition, the self-organizing chemical reaction will eventually settle down in one of the two patterns. Therefore, there is no ambiguity of the situation at hand. Let us turn next to seemingly ambiguous situations of the visual world. This is illustrated in Figure 3B in terms of the spinning dancer paradigm (but applies to all kinds of seemingly perceptual ambiguities such as discussed in the context of the Necker cube or the MIB phenomenon). The spinning dancer movie creates external circumstances such that the whole system composed of the human observer and the external circumstances represent a self-organizing system that features a certain symmetry property. The system can exhibit two kinds of brain activity patterns: one pattern related to the percept of a clockwise spinning dancer, the other pattern related to the percept of a counter-clockwise spinning dancer. In what follows brain activity patterns will be described in terms of firing rates of spatially distributed neuron populations. In Figure 3B a group of four neuron populations is considered. Two possible firing rates patterns are illustrated qualitatively (where full circles, circles with a bar, and empty circles stand for high, medium, and low firing rates). These patterns denote the reaction of the brain to the spinning dancer movie and for this reason are referred to as brain activity reaction patterns. Note that the brain activity patterns are shown in Figure 3 for illustration purposes only. The firing rates have been chosen arbitrarily and do not reflect any experimental data. Due to the assumed symmetry of the perceptual system exposed to the dancer movie both patterns can emerge. The two patterns correspond to reaction patterns that have similarities to brain activity patterns that would emerge if the individual under consideration is viewing a clockwise (CW) or a counter-clockwise (CCW) rotating object. Again it is assumed that both patterns are competitive such that only one pattern can emerge at a time. Which pattern emerges depends on the initial conditions given in terms of the brain activity at the beginning of the experiment. Therefore, the system is not ambiguous. We see that although the phrase "perceptual ambiguity" is frequently used in the literature, from a self-organization perspective the correct phrase of the situation at hand is "perceptual bistability".

The self-organization perspective as such explains the emergence of a pattern and in our context the emergence of the percept of a rotating dancer. In order to address oscillatory perception, we need to add a second component to the theoretical framework: a feedback or self-regulation mechanism (Haken, 1991). In order to do so, we distinguish between processes taking place on two different time scales. Accordingly, the pattern formation process is assumed to take place on a relatively fast time scale. The neuronal activity evolving on that fast time scale describes the so-called active state of the system. The dynamics of the fast evolving brain activity is determined by the structure of the neuronal network. The structure of the neuronal network is assumed to be almost constant on the time scale of the pattern formation process. However, when the same percept is perceived for a longer period, the structure is assumed to change slowly. Therefore, the structural features of the neuronal network correspond from a mathematical perspective to time-dependent variables that vary on a time scale that is slow relative to the variables of the active state. Importantly, the changes on the slow time scale can break the symmetry property of the system and create a bias. More precisely, consistent with the observed perceptual oscillations, it is plausible to assume that a percept inhibits itself. Therefore, after a certain duration, the bistable system becomes monostable such that only the alternative percept is stable. For example, if the dancer is perceived as rotating clockwise, then the percept of the clockwise rotating dancer is inhibited and eventually becomes unstable. As a result, the brain activity pattern related to the clockwise rotating dancer disappears and the alternative brain activity pattern of the counter-clockwise rotating dancer emerges. The active state and the structure constitute the whole perceptual system of interest. The two components taken together are referred to as grand state, see Figure 4 (panel A). As illustrated in Figure 4A, the two components mutually depend on each other, which leads to the phenomenon of oscillatory perception. A given pattern of brain activity affects the structure such that it inhibits its emergence (see panel B). Due to mutual competition between the brain activity patterns under consideration (see panel B), the pattern becomes unstable and the alternative pattern emerges. Then the process repeats itself. Finally, note that from a mechanistic perspective, the active state may correspond to firing rates of neuron populations, while the structure may correspond to synaptic weights connecting different neuron populations.

The mathematical details of the neuronal network model have been worked out in several studies (Ditzinger et al., 1989, Frank, 2014; Haken, 1991). In what follows, we will use the model proposed by Frank (2014) because it allows for a semi-analytical treatment and is based on the Lotka-Volterra-Haken model for self-organization (Frank, 2016).

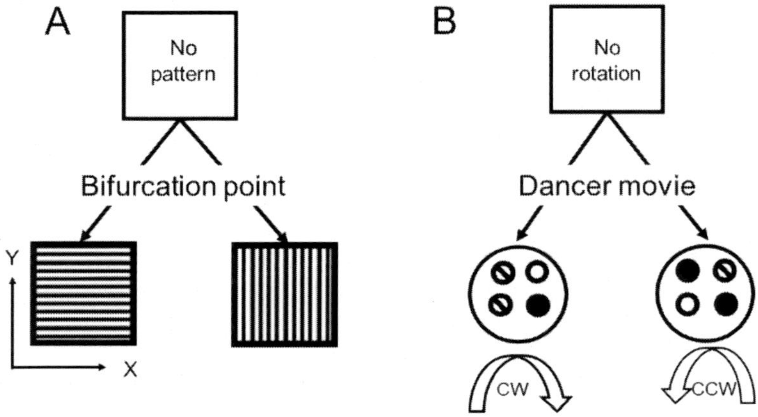

Figure 3. Explanation of the symmetry hypothesis. Panel A: Symmetric design of chemical systems leads to bistability of chemical stripe patterns. Panel B: Structural symmetry of neuronal networks is assumed to lead to perceptual bistability in the spinning dancer paradigm. Large circles with four components illustrate schematically two different brain activity patterns. The four components illustrate qualitatively different firing rates of four neuron populations. The patterns are shown for illustration purposes only. The explicit patterns are irrelevant and are not related to any experimental data. CW: clockwise. CCW: counter-clockwise.

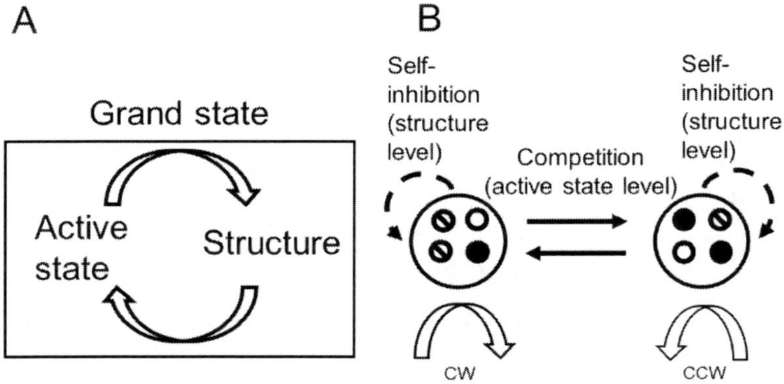

Figure 4. Overview of levels and interactions of the neuronal network under consideration. Panel A: Active state and structure constitute the grand state and interact with each other. Panel B: Key interactions determining the dynamics of the spinning dancer neuronal network. The self-inhibition loops and the competitive interaction mechanism are shown.

The Lotka-Volterra-Haken neuronal network model exhibits two levels: a pattern and amplitude level. Accordingly, a pattern of brain activity is described by a spatial layout of firing rates over a certain area of the brain. This layout is referred to as basis pattern. The basis pattern is weighted by a variable, which is called the pattern amplitude. That is, all firing rates of the layout (basis pattern) are weighted in the same way by the pattern amplitude. The pattern amplitude is bounded by zero on the one hand and a saturation value on the other hand. If a pattern amplitude equals zero or is relatively small (as compared to pattern amplitudes of alternative patterns), then the pattern is absent. In contrast, if the amplitude is close to its saturation value, then the pattern is present. As such, different patterns may be present at the same time, which is called co-existence of patterns. However, in what follows, we will consider the case of mutually exclusive patterns. This implies that only one pattern can emerge at a time. The network exhibits a "winner-takes-all" dynamics (Haken, 1991). Figure 5 shows simulation results of the Lotka-Volterra-Haken amplitude equation model. Panel A shows the evolution of the pattern amplitudes of the CW and CCW basis patterns. The amplitudes are continuous variables and accordingly increase and decrease in a more or less smooth fashion. In contrast, panel C describes the brain activity in terms of three discrete states. Either the CW or CCW pattern is present or both patterns are absent. In the latter case, we may say that the individual under consideration perceives "nothing" in the sense that he or she has no perception of a rotation direction. Comparing panels A and C, we see that the CW and CCW patterns are assumed to be present when their amplitudes are close to their corresponding saturation values (Frank, 2009). As mentioned above, the underlying mechanism for perceptual oscillation involves self-inhibition that acts on the structure of the neuronal network. To account for this mechanism, the amplitude dynamics is supplemented with a dynamics of structural parameters. These parameters have also been called growth parameters (Frank, 2015, 2016). From mathematical point of view they corresponds to eigenvalues. A key feature of the pattern formation approach is that each basis pattern feature its own structural parameter. The evolution of the structural parameters for the CW and CCW patterns is shown in panel B. In line with our previous discussion, the structural parameter of a pattern that is present decays as long as the pattern is present. Due to this attenuation of the structural parameters of emerged patterns, patterns become eventually (i.e., at certain values of the structural parameters) unstable. The brain activity dynamics makes a transition to the alternative pattern. The consequences of this switch or transition are twofold. First, the structural parameter of the pattern that just disappeared increases again towards its baseline level. Second, the structural parameter of the pattern that has just emerged begins to decay due to the self-inhibition mechanism. If the structural parameter of the absent basis pattern has increased to a sufficiently large value relative to the parameter of the present basis pattern, then the present basis pattern becomes unstable. The cycle composed of two basis patterns is completed and a new cycle begins.

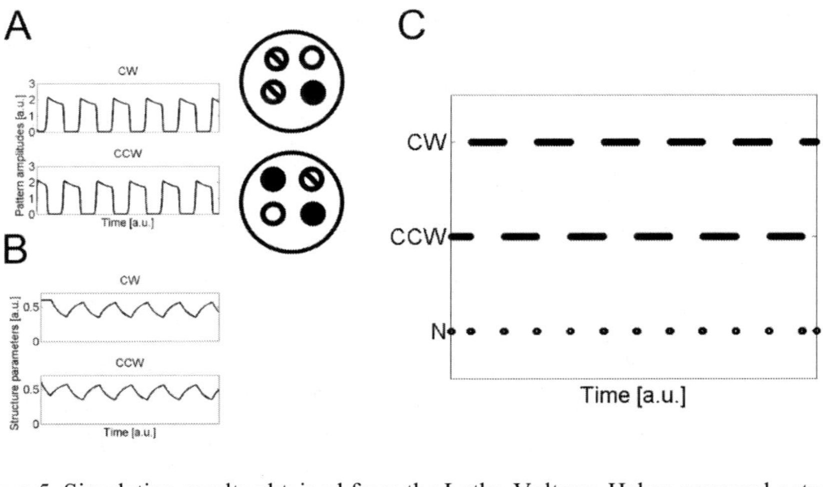

Figure 5. Simulation results obtained from the Lotka-Volterra-Haken neuronal network (Frank, 2014, 2016). Panel A: Pattern amplitudes of the brain activity reaction patterns to clockwise (CW) and counter-clockwise (CCW) object rotations as functions of time. Panel B: Evolution of the corresponding structural parameters shown on the same time scale as the amplitude dynamics. Panel C: Temporal sequence of categorical brain states as obtained from the amplitude dynamics shown in panel A. For details see Frank (2014, 2016).

General Discussion

This section is composed of two parts. First, we will discuss the experimental findings reported above in the context of the Lotka-Volterra-Haken neuronal network model. Second, we will discuss a number of fundamental issues that have been pointed out in the literature in the context of oscillatory perception of seemingly ambiguous situations.

As reported above, in the context of the spinning dancer experiment, it was found that the focus of individuals affects the rate of perceptual switches. Consequently, it is assumed that there is an interaction between the brain activity patterns describing the focus of an individual and the aforementioned oscillatory brain activity dynamics induced by seemingly ambivalent circumstances. Figure 6 provides details of this neuropsychological perspective. It is assumed that when individuals focus on the lower or upper part of the dancer movie, then these activities are related on the neuronal level to two different brain activity patterns. Without loss of generality, these activity patterns are illustrated in panel A by means of a group of three neuron populations. These focus-related brain activity patterns are assumed to impact directly or indirectly the structure of the neuronal oscillatory system. That is, the focus-related brain activity patterns may push (direct impact) the structure parameters to low or high levels. Alternatively, the forces elicited by the spinning dancer movie and acting on the human brain via the visual system differ across the two focus conditions. This in turn may imply that the structural parameters of the neuronal oscillator operate on different baseline levels. It can be shown that the oscillation frequency (i.e., the switching rate) increases as a function of the magnitude of the structural parameters. Therefore, the postulated direct or indirect impact of the focus-related brain activity patterns is such that the upper-body focus brain activity pattern leads to relative small structural parameters, whereas the lower-body focus brain activity pattern yields relative large structural parameters, see panel A. The structural parameters determine the frequency of the switches between the brain activity reaction patterns of the CW and CCW rotating objects, see bottom part of panel A. Panels B and C show simulation results for the averaged structural parameters of low and high level shown in panel A. For the low-magnitude parameters the periods between the switches are long and, consequently, the switching rate is low. In contrast, for high-magnitude structural parameters the periods between switches are short and the switching rate is high.

Let us turn next to the observation of a transient phase. That is, we observed that in block 2 the switching rate was higher than in block 1. This result can be interpreted in terms of an adaptation mechanism that acts on a time scale of minutes. In this context, Figure 7 demonstrates two hypotheses. According to the first hypothesis, it is assumed that during block 1 the emerging brain activity patterns affects the structure of the oscillatory neuronal network such that the structure parameters (eigenvalues) that determine the oscillation frequency increase gradually. More precisely, as illustrated in the top half of Figure 7, the first hypothesis assumes that the transient phase phenomenon is caused by a circular causality loop. On the one hand, the neuronal network structure determines the switching rate between the two basis patterns that are reactions to CW and CCW rotating objects. On the other hand, the emerging patterns modify the structure of the network by increasing the structure parameters. This first hypothesis involves higher cognitive brain functioning. In contrast, the second hypothesis assumes that the transient phase is due to lower level brain functioning, that is, processes in the early steps of visual perception. Accordingly, the dancer movie, irrespective of the emerging brain activity reaction patterns, affects the neuronal network by increasing its structural parameters (eigenvalues). Importantly, both hypotheses attempt to clarify that time as such is not the cause for the observed increase of the switching rate. That is, although from an experimental design perspective, time was the independent variable of the experiment, from a mechanistic perspective, we hypothesize that either the dancer movie (i.e., the forces acting on the brain) or the emerging brain activity patterns (i.e., the reactions of the brain to the forces) caused the observed increase of the switching rate across to two experimental blocks.

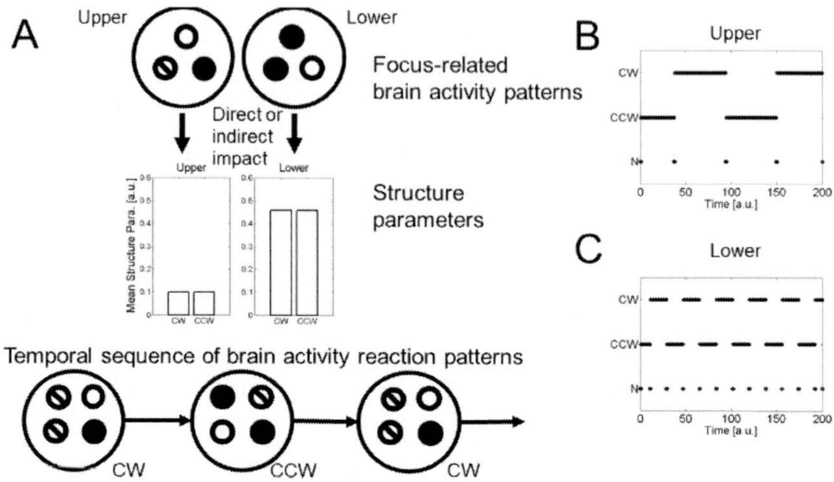

Figure 6. Interpretation of the main effect of focus on the switching rate observed in the spinning dancer experiment in terms of the Lotka-Volterra-Haken neuronal network model. See text for details.

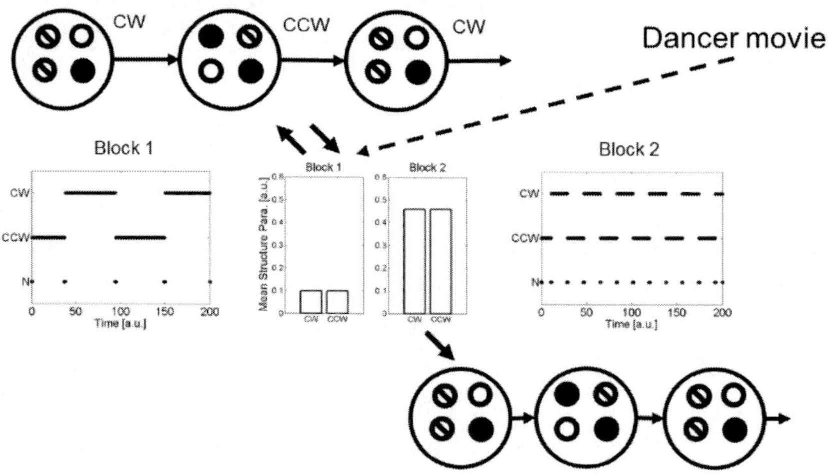

Figure 7. Interpretation of the main effect of time on the switching rate observed in the spinning dancer experiment in terms of the Lotka-Volterra-Haken neuronal network model. See text for details.

Finally, let us re-interpret our results from the MIB experiment in the context of the Lotka-Volterra-Haken neuronal network oscillator model. In line with previous work (Bonneh et al., 2001), we observed that the number of disappearances per time unit increased, when the background rotation speed was increased. In the context of the MIB experiment, the Lotka-Volterra-Haken model describes switches between brain activity reaction patterns to complete and incomplete three-dots triangles in front of a rotating background. Although the brain activity patterns of incomplete three-dots triangles form a class of patterns, previous work has shown that formally they can be regarded as a single pattern (Frank, 2014). Therefore, from a modeling perspective we are concerned with switches between two patterns: the pattern related to the complete three-dots triangle and a pattern that stands for the class of patterns related to incomplete three-dots triangles. Figure 8 illustrates the application of the Lotka-Volterra-Haken model to the MIB experiment. In panel A (bottom part) a temporal sequence composed of two brain activity reaction patterns is shown. The two patterns are only qualitatively described. Without loss of generality, they are described by means of the firing rates of a group of five neuron populations. The first pattern is assumed to have similarity with a pattern that would emerge if an individual is exposed to a complete three-dots triangle irrespective of the background. Consequently, if this first pattern emerges in the context of the MIB experiment, then this means that the complete three-dots triangle is perceived in front of the moving background. In contrast, the second pattern stands for all patterns that have similarities to patterns induced by incomplete variants of the three-dots triangle. As sketched in panel A (bottom part) the two brain activity patterns emerge and disappear in an alternating fashion. The frequency of the switches between the patterns is determined by the structural properties of the oscillatory perceptual neuronal network. As mentioned above, the Lotka-Volterra-Haken network exhibits particular structural parameters (eigenvalues) that determine the switching rate. In line with the observed impact of the background rotation speed on the switching frequency, it is assumed that rotation speed affects those structural parameters. The parameters (eigenvalues) increase in magnitude as rotation speed increases, see panel A. Simulation results are shown in panels B,C and D. For small, medium, and large structural parameters simulations of the model yield low-frequency (B), medium-frequency (C), and high-frequency (D) switching sequences between the patterns. This is tantamount to say that for slow, medium, and fast background rotations the model yields alternating sequences with low (B), medium (C), and high (D) switching rates.

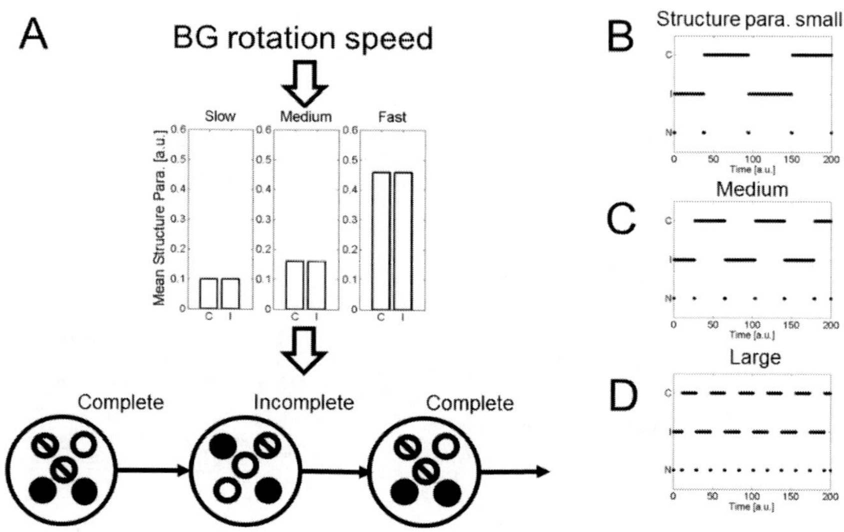

Figure 8. Interpretation of the speed effect of the number of disappearances (and consequently the switching rate between complete and incomplete percepts) observed in the motion-induced blindness experiment in terms of the Lotka-Volterra-Haken neuronal network model. See text for details.

In this second part of the discussion section, we would like to address some special topics related to the phenomenon of perceptual oscillations induced by seemingly ambiguous circumstances of the visual world. First of all, as pointed out above, ambiguities do not exist. Rather, circumstances may give rise to multistable perceptual systems and multistable neuronal networks in particular. The main point to be made here is that human behavior, cognition, and perception in general is deterministic (Skinner, 1953). That is, to a good approximation, human behavior follows deterministic laws that can be formulated in terms of evolution equations of dynamical systems (such as the amplitude equations of the Lotka-Volterra-Haken model). The same holds for cognition and perception. The scientific approach to understand the human nature is based (or by definition implies) the notion that there is no arbitrariness or free will. Note that this general point of view also holds if stochastic aspects (e.g., randomness) are taken into consideration. Humans are considered as bio-machines (Skinner, 1953) that satisfy laws and behave according to those laws just as engineered machines (cell phones, coffee makers, cars, etc.) satisfy laws and "behave" accordingly. In order to emphasis this point, let us return to the basic question about the rotation direction of the spinning dancer. We have argued above that the answer to the question "in which direction does the silhouetted dancer rotate?" depends on the initial active state of the individual who is watching the movie. According to the neuronal network model, the initial state of the brain activity determines which rotation direction is initially perceived. For example, if the individual exhibits a brain activity pattern that exhibits great similarity to brain activity reaction patterns of clockwise rotating objects, then the individual will initially perceive the dancer as rotating clockwise. Figure 9 illustrates this point. Figure 9 shows a so-called phase portrait of the amplitude dynamics of the Lotka-Volterra-Haken neuronal network model assuming that the structure parameters (eigenvalues) do not change with time. This is a good approximation for the period in which an individual is exposed for the very first time to the movie. It is also assumed that the neuronal network exhibit perfect symmetry. The phase portrait shows how the amplitudes evolve in the space spanned by the two amplitudes of the CW and CCW basis patterns. Full dots represent the end points of the amplitude dynamics. They correspond to the emergence of the CW brain activity pattern (dot on the horizontal axis) and CCW brain activity pattern (dot on the vertical axis), respectively. The end points feature the saturation values of the respective amplitudes. The open circles denote unstable points at which the amplitude dynamics does not change over time. However, they cannot be reached due to their unstable nature. Figure 9 illustrates that the space spanned by the two amplitudes is separated by the diagonal (dashed line) into two halves. The top-left half is the basis of attraction for the CCW brain activity pattern. That is, if the initial brain activity of an individual is such that it falls in this region, then the CCW pattern will emerge and an individual will perceive the dancer as rotating counter-clockwise. In contrast, if the initial brain activity of an individual correspond to a point in the lower-right half region, then the CW pattern will emerge and the individual will perceive the dancer as rotating clockwise. Note that from a mathematical point of view, the amplitudes can be larger than their respective saturation values. The region in the two-dimensional plane with amplitudes larger than their saturation values typically cannot be approached. However, due to the fact that the structure parameters (eigenvalues) of the network in general are assumed to vary, it is possible that initial values assume larger than saturation values.

While the theory of self-organization explains the emergence of brain activity patterns at a bifurcation point, it cannot explain why the system approaches the bifurcation point at all. Therefore, a two-tiered model was proposed above. Tier 1 and 2 correspond to active state and structure, respectively. Accordingly, we assumed that the brain activity in terms of active state dynamics (tier 1) affects structural brain properties (tier 2). These structural properties in turn determine the active state brain dynamics. In order to distinguish between the two tiers it was assumed that the active state dynamics evolves on a time scale that is fast relative to the dynamics of the structural properties. In particular, we assumed that emerging patterns inhibit the circumstance on the structural level that supported their emergence in the first place. The self-inhibition proposal echoes various suggestions that have been made earlier in the literature.

To begin with, various authors have suggested that the repeated switching between percepts induced by seemingly ambiguous pictures is a consequence of neuronal fatigue (Horlitz and O'Leary, 1993; Koehler 1940; Mueller et al., 1999). The notion of fatigue implies some kind of effort. In the context of the Lotka-Volterra-Haken model, the effort would be the build-up of brain activity reaction patterns. In summary, the emergence of a self-organized brain activity patterns may be regarded as an effort, while the decay of a structure parameter (eigenvalue) may be interpreted as fatigue caused by this effort.

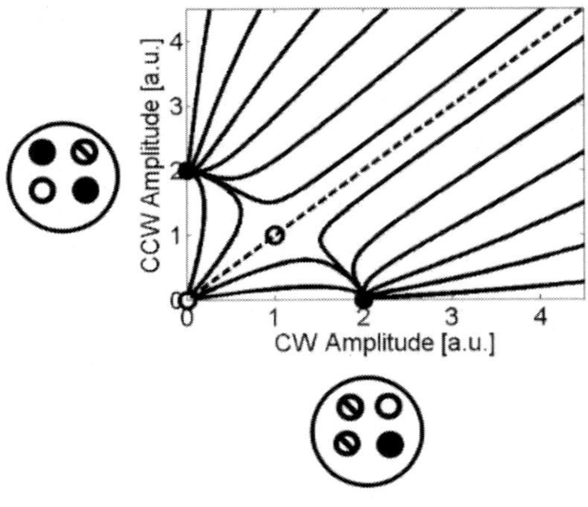

Figure 9. Phase portrait of the amplitude equations of the Lotka-Volterra-Haken model for the symmetric case in case of the spinning dancer paradigm. The amplitudes of the brain activity reaction patterns to counter-clockwise (CCW) and clockwise (CW) rotating objects are plotted against each other in the same two-dimensional plane for different time points. Full dots denote stable end points of the dynamics and correspond to the emergence of either of the two possible brain activity reaction patterns. See text for details.

Another theoretical account consistent with our proposed model is inhibition theory. Inhibition theory (among other things) states that the performance of a mental task inhibits the performed task. That is, it is assumed that there is an inhibition variable that increases during the performance of the task. Importantly, it is not time but the task performance, which causes the inhibition variable to increase. Therefore, the inhibition is also called reactive inhibition. Inhibition theory has been applied to explain perceptual oscillations due to perceptual rivalry (Van der Ven et al., 2005).

A third phenomenon consistent with our modeling approach is the inhibition of return effect (Klein, 2000; Posner et al., 1985). The effect is found for example in visual search experiments. Roughly speaking, when a target object pops up repeatedly in a given area and a test person searches for that target, then the time to find the object is relatively short when the object shows up at different locations. In contrast, when the object is shown at the same location at which it occurred in the previous instance, then the time to find the object in the second trial is relatively long. In other words, individuals have the tendency not search at the same place twice. To return to the same search location is inhibited, whence the name "inhibition of return". From a neurophysiological perspective, it has been suggested that there is an inhibitory feedback loop that reduces the foreground property of the target if it occurs a second time at the same location (Posner et al., 1985; Prime and Ward, 2006). This neurophysiological explanation has in common with our proposed model that the perception of something at a given moment in time inhibits that the same perceptual process happens again at a later moment in time.

As mentioned in the introduction, neurophysiological experimental studies have been conducted with humans and monkeys to investigate repetitively switching in the context of the Necker cube paradigm (Britz et al., 2009; Kornmeier et al., 2004), perceptual rivalry (Leopold et al., 1999; Sterzer et al., 2009), and the apparent motion paradigm (Mueller et al., 1999, 2005). Although these studies were not tailored to address predictions of self-organization approaches such as given in terms of the Lotka-Volterra-Haken neuronal network model, in closing this section let us re-interpret the basic finding of these studies in the context of the aforementioned modeling efforts. The rationale of the aforementioned neurophysiological experimental studies was to identify brain activity that is characteristic for the switching between percepts. That is, according to the researchers of those studies, there are differences between the periods in which no switching occurs and the periods in which switching happens. In contrast, the self-organization perspective states that there is a temporal alternating sequence of different brain activity reaction patterns that are experienced as different percepts. In order to unify these two perspectives, let us have a closer look at the transitions between brain activity patterns as predicted by the Lotka-Volterra-Haken model.

Let us address the amplitude variables first (i.e., the active state). As shown in Figure 5 (panel A) at switching points one amplitude variable drops from its saturation value to zero, while the alternative amplitude increases sharply from zero to its saturation value. This implies that during the switching periods there are dramatic changes of brain activity, whereas during periods in which no switching occurs brain activity changes only slightly. Mathematically speaking, if we consider the amplitude time-derivatives (i.e., changes of the amplitudes over time) rather than the amplitudes themselves, then during perceptual switches there is a great amount of activity in these amplitude time-derivative measures, whereas during periods of constant perception the activity is relatively low. If neurophysiological measurements are sensitive to those amplitude time-derivative measures then our model would predict the fundamental observation that was made in the aforementioned experimental studies.

Second, let us address the structural variables (i.e., the structure level). As shown in panel B of Figure 5, the structure parameters (e.g., given in terms of synaptic weights) vary in an oscillatory fashion. They do so close to switching points and far away from switching points. Therefore, at first sight, on the structural level the switching and non-switching periods seem not to feature different characteristic properties. However, the mathematical model used to describe the evolution of the structure parameters has been chosen for simplicity and parsimony purposes. It is not intended to fit any experimental data. Any monotonically decaying or increasing functions can be used. Therefore, a dynamics of the structure parameters that looks quite differently can qualitatively yield the same results as presented above but fit better experimental results. In particular, we may imagine a temporal evolution of the structure parameters (eigenvalues) that is relatively constant over long time periods but exhibits dramatic changes at the switching points. Such a dynamics would be consistent with the experimental findings of the aforementioned experimental studies assuming that the neurophysiologic measurements of the experimental studies picked up brain activity related to processes that lead to changes in the connections between neuron populations (i.e., processes of plasticity changing the synaptic weights).

References

Attneave, F. (1971). Multistability in perception. *Scientific American*, *225*, 63-71.

Bonneh, Y. S., Cooperman, A. & Sagi, D. (2001). Motion-induced blindness in normal observers. *Nature*, *411*, 798-801.

Borsellino, A., De Maroc, A., Allazetta, A., Rinesi, S. & Bartollini, B. (1972). Reversal time distribution in the perception of visual ambiguous stimuli. *Kybernetik*, *10*, 139-144.

Britz, J., Landis, T. & Michel, C. M. (2009). Right parietal brain activity precedes perceptual alternation of bistable stimuli. *Cerebral Cortex*, *19*, 55-65.

Carter, O. L. & Pettigrew, J. D. (2003). A common oscillator for perceptual rivalries. *Perception*, *32*, 295-305.

Ditzinger, T. & Haken, H. (1989). Oscillations in perception and ambiguous patterns. *Biological Cybernetics*, *61*, 279-287.

Frank, T. D. (2009). On a multistable competitive network model in the case of an inhomogeneous growth rate spectrum: with an application to priming. *Physics Letters A*, *373*, 4127-4133.

Frank, T. D. (2014). Multistable perception in schizophrenia: a model-based analysis via coarse-grained order parameter dynamics and a comment on the fourth law. *Universal Journal of Psychology*, *2*, 231-240.

Frank, T. D. (2015). On the interplay between order parameter dynamics and system parameter dynamics in human perceptual-cognitive-behavioral systems. *Nonlinear Dynamics, Psychology, and Life Sciences*, *19*, 111-146.

Frank, T. D. (2016). Perception adapts via top-down regulation to task repetition: a Lotka-Volterra-Haken modeling analysis of experimental data. *Journal of Integrative Neuroscience*, *15*, 67-79.

Goldstein, E. B. (2010). *Sensation and Perception*. Belmont, CA: Wadsworth.

Haken, H. (1991). *Synergetic computers and cognition*. Berlin: Springer.

Haken, H. (1996). *Principles of brain functioning*. Berlin: Springer.

Horlitz, K. L. & O'Leary, A. (1993). Satiation or availability? Effects of attention, memory and imagery on the perception of ambiguous figures. *Perception and Psychophysics, 53*, 668-681.

Kelso, J. A. S. (1995). *Dynamic patterns: the self-organization of brain and behavior.* Cambridge: MIT Press.

Klein, R. M. (2000). Inhibition of return. *Trends in Cognitive Science, 4*, 138-147.

Kornmeier, J. & Bach, M. (2004). Early neural activity in Necker-cube reversal: evidence for low-level processing of a gestalt phenomenon. *Psychophysiology*, *41*, 1-8.

Kornmeier, J., Hein C. M. & Bach, M. (2009). Multistable perception. when bottom-up and top-down coincide. *Brian and Cognition*, *69*, 138-147.

Koehler, W. (1940). *Dynamics in Psychology*. New York: Liveright.

Liu, C. H., Tzeng, O. J. L., Hung, D. L., Tseng, P. & Juan, C. H. (2012). Investigation of bistable perception with the silhouette spinner: sit still, spin the dancer with your will. *Vision Research*, *60*, 34-39.

Leopold, D. A. & Logothetis, N. K. (1999). Multistable phenomena: changing views in perception. *Trends in Cognitive Sciences*, *3*, 255-264.

Posner, M. I., Rafak, R. D., Choate, L. S. & Vaughan, J. (1985). Inhibition of return: neural basis and function. *Cognitive Neuropsychology*, *2*, 211-228.

Prime, D. J. & Ward, L. M. (2006). Cortical expressions of inhibition of return. *Brain Research*, *1072*, 161-174.

Mamassian, P. & Landy, M. S. (1998). Observer biases in the 3D interpretation of line drawings. *Vision Research*, *38*, 2817-2832.

Mamassian, P. & Goutcher, R. (2005). Temporal dynamics in bistable perception. *Journal of Vision*, *5*, 361-375.

Mueller, T. J., Federspiel, A., Fallgatter, A. J. & Strik, W. K. (1999). EEG signs of vigilance fluctuations preceding perceptual flips in multistable illusionary motion. *Neuroreport*, *10*, 3423-3427.

Mueller, T. J., Koenig, T., Wackermann, J., Kalus, P., Fallgatter, A., Strik, W. & Lehmann, D. (2005). Subsecond changes of global brain state in illusory multistable motion perception. *Journal of Neural Transmission*, *112*, 565-576.

Pettigrew, J. D. (2001). Searching for the switch: neural basis for perceptual rivalry alternations. *Brain and Mind*, *2*, 85-118.

Skinner, B. F. (1953). *Science and human behavior*. New York: The Free Press.

Sheppard, B. M. & Pettigrew, J. D. (2006). Plaid motion rivalry: correlates with binocular rivalry and positive mood state. *Perception*, *35*, 157-169.

Sterzer, P., Kleinschmidt, A. & Rees, G. (2009). The neural basis of multistable perception. *Trends in Cognitive Science*, *13*, 311-318.

Van der Ven, A. H. G. S., Gremmen, F. M. & Smit, J. C. (2005). A statistical model for binocular rivalry. *British Journal of Mathematical and Statistical Psychology*, *58*, 97-116.

In: Horizons in Neuroscience Research ISBN: 978-1-53613-286-1
Editors: A. Costa and E. Villalba

Chapter 3

THE NEUROBIOLOGICAL ASPECTS OF EXPOSURE TO CHILDHOOD MALTREATMENT

Arta Dodaj[1], PhD, Kristina Sesar[2], PhD and Nataša Šimić[1], PhD

[1]Department of Psychology, University of Zadar, Zadar, Croatia

[2]Centre of Mental Health, Široki Brijeg, Bosnia and Herzegovina

ABSTRACT

Childhood maltreatment is the most frequent form of trauma during early childhood, which may cause numerous difficulties, both in childhood and in adulthood. This chapter gives an overview of research so far into the effect of maltreatment in childhood on structural and functional changes to various parts of the nervous system. In people exposed to maltreatment in childhood numerous neurobiological changes have been found, primarily in the neuroendocrine systems activated by stress, which include the function of the autonomous nervous system, and the hypothalamic–pituitary–adrenal axis. The consequences of maltreatment in childhood are also evident in the prefrontal cortex region of the brain, as well as in various parts of the limbic system. Research also reports the negative effects of maltreatment on the development of the corpus callosum. The results of research so far indicate that when studying the effect of traumatic experience, such as maltreatment in childhood, the many factors involved must not be overlooked, such as the developmental period when the maltreatment occurred, the child's sex, and the severity and form of maltreatment to which the child was exposed. These factors separately, but also their interactive effects, may change the mechanism of the effects of maltreatment on neurobiological processes.

Keywords: biological stress system, brain development, child maltreatment

1. Introduction

According to the World Health Organization (2002), maltreatment in childhood is defined as physical abuse, emotional abuse, sexual abuse, neglect or exploitation of a child, that results in actual or potential harm to the child's health, survival, development or dignity. In more recent times, witnessing family violence has also been recognized as a form of abusive behaviour, which affects the child's health and safety, but also their psychological development (Delima & Vimpani, 2011; Kitzmann, Gaylord, Holt, & Kenny, 2003; Levendosky, Bogat, & Martinez-Torteya, 2013). The consequences of expose to abuse and neglect in childhood are not the same for all children. For some children and young people the consequences may be chronic, whilst others may experience less unfavourable outcomes (Miller-Perrin & Perrin, 2007). Family circumstances and other positive or negative experiences in life affect the child's development and their resilience in facing abuse. The critical factors which affect the consequences which maltreatment and neglect may have for a child or young person are the frequency and duration of the maltreatment, and the exposure to different forms of chronic maltreatment. Chronic abuse is deemed to be repeated episodes of abuse over a prolonged period of time (Bromfield & Higgins, 2005). Research confirms that exposure to various forms of abuse, that is, multiple maltreatment, has more serious consequences than exposure to only one form of abuse (Finkelhor, Ormrod, Turner, & Hamby, 2005; Higgins & McCabe, 2001; Ethier, Lemelin, &Lacharite, 2004; Graham et al., 2010; Johnson-Reid, Kohl, & Brett, 2012), which is actually very rare. In an attempt to explain some of the negative consequences related to chronic and multiple abuses, the term "complex trauma" is often used. This term relates to multiple symptoms which include a wide range of cognitive, affective and behavioural consequences related to prolonged trauma, especially if the traumatic events occur early in childhood (Price-Robertson, Rush, Wall, & Higgins, 2013). Complex trauma has serious consequences for the development of the child's brain, which is still developing in that phase of life. It may hinder the child's ability to integrate sensory, emotional and cognitive information, which may lead to excessive reactions to stress, and long-term consequences, such as various physical, cognitive, behavioural and other psychological sequelae (Streeck-Fischer & van der Kolk, 2000).

The human brain develops intensively in the period of early childhood. In order to understand the changes in its development in unfavourable circumstances for development, such as abuse and neglect, an understanding is necessary of brain development in an optimal, stimulating environment. Its development should be seen as a continuous process, from the initial organogenesis in the prenatal period, up until adulthood. In the first five years of life the volume of the brain increases in connection with the development of white matter and the differentiation of grey matter. However, from the 7th to the 17th year of life, the white matter increases progressively due to myelination processes, whilst the grey matter is mainly un-differentiated, and the total size of the brain does not change significantly (Casey, Giedd, &Thomas, 2000; Durstonet al., 2001; Giedd, Blumenthal, & Jeffries, 1999; Paus et al., 1999). Regarding the grey matter, in this period differentiation primarily takes place in the regions of the frontal and parietal lobes of the cerebral cortex (Rapoportet al., 1999; Sowell et al., 1999). The basal ganglia shrink is size, whilst the corpus callosum (Gieddet al., 1999; Thompson et al., 2000), the hippocampus and the amygdala (Gieddet al., 1996; Giedd, Castellanos, Rajapakse, Vaituzis, & Rapoport, 1997; Pfefferbaumet al., 1994) increase in size. The total mass of the brain is 10% greater in boys than in girls (Gielddet al., 1996). In young adults and adults, that is from 20 to 70 years of age, the caudate nucleus (Jernigan et al., 1991), the area of the diencephalon gradually shrink (Jernigan et al., 1991) and in general the differentiation of the grey matter is reduced (Jernigan et al., 1991; Sullivan, Marsh, Mathalon, Lim, & Pfefferbaum, 1995). In this period, the reduced differentiation of the grey matter is particularly intense in the temporal and frontal lobes of the cerebral cortex (Jernigan et al., 1991; Sullivan et al., 1995). Researchers also report the change in width of the chambers of the brain during childhood development (Jernigan et al., 1991; Sullivan et al., 1995). On the basis of all this, but also other documented changes that take place during the development of the brain, it can be expected that exposure to negative experiences in different periods of life will result in deviations in its development.

As has already been said, different parts of the brain develop and are organized intensively precisely during childhood. For a child to have normal neuro-motor and psychological development in the period of early and late childhood a stimulating environment is vital, that is, one which provides the possibility of learning, exploration and experimentation, and getting to know the surrounding world. Exposure to various negative circumstances, however, may lead to a number of abnormalities in neurobiological development (van der Kolk, 2003), which in the end may result in the risk of the development of various psychological symptoms in puberty and/or adulthood (Teicheret al., 2003).

In the past few decades, there has been a great deal of interest shown in research aimed at examining the changes to different parts of the nervous system affected by traumatic experiences, including changes in the function of various neurotransmitter systems, as well as atypical or abnormal hormonal reactions etc. (Bremner, 2006). With the development of techniques for visualization and detection of signals from various parts of the brain, it has become possible to gain a detailed insight into changes caused by early trauma in childhood (French, 2008). The purpose of this chapter is to present the results of research undertaken so far on the influence of abuse in childhood on the development and function of various parts of the nervous system.

2. Maltreatment and Neuro-Endocrine Systems Activated by Stress

2.1. The Effect of Maltreatment in Childhood on the Function of the Autonomous Nervous System

In stressful situations, the activation increases of the sympathetic nervous system, which has an important role in the reaction of the organism, mobilizing its energy reserves. "Mobilization" here actually means preparation of the organism for defence, and is seen in an increase in pulse rate, increased blood pressure, rapid breathing, stimulation of the sweat glands, the halting or deceleration of the digestive system, and similar reactions. The increased reaction of the sympathetic nervous system is connected to fear and anxiety, and it also indicates a strong emotional response in the individual (Murray-Close, Holland, & Roisman, 2012). Recovery from stress is also accompanied by the relevant wandering nerve, which promotes a calming effect, stimulating the release of prolactin, vasopressin and oxytocin (Cornwall, 2016). People with a strong response to this para-sympathetic nerve recover quickly from stress (according to Porges, 2009).

Research shows that in persons exposed to maltreatment in childhood, at the time of an induced stressful event, there is hyperactivity of the autonomous nervous system, which is linked to increased arousal of the organism and repeated experience of the trauma (Bryant, Harvey, Gurhtie, & Moulds, 2000; Heim, Ehlert, & Hellhammer, 2000a). In them, the increased activation of the sympathetic nervous system is most often seen in raised blood pressure and increased pulse rate (Heim et al., 2000b; Lorenz, Harte, & Meston, 2015).

2.2. The Effect of Exposure to Maltreatment in Childhood on the Function of the Hypothalamic–Pituitary–Adrenal Axis

Many studies of various traumatic and stressful experiences have been aimed at examining the function of the hypothalamic–pituitary–adrenal axis (HPA) and measuring glucocorticoids and their final products. Exposure to trauma causes a number of changes in the function of this system, which is important for maintaining the biological balance of the organism in normal circumstances, but especially in stressful situations (Cook, Ciorciari, Varker, & Devilly, 2009; De Bellis, 2007; De Bellis et al., 1999; Tarullo & Gunnar, 2006). The HPA axis reaches maturity in its function at the age of 4 years (van Goozen, Fairchild, Snoek, & Harold, 2007). Its origin is in the paraventricular nucleus of the hypothalamus, which, through the corticotropin-releasing hormone, prompts the adenohypophysis (pituitary gland) to increase production of the adrenocorticotropic hormone (ACTH). Increased production of ACTH prompts the release of glucocorticoids, especially cortisol, from the adrenal glands. Cortisol is the main glucocorticoid, which is also known as the stress hormone, because it prompts the mobilization of energy and helps the organism to combat stress (Disseth, 2005). In research it is used as a measurement of stress levels, and conclusions are drawn about the dysregulation of the HPA axis on the basis of monitoring its concentrations in the blood or saliva. It has been confirmed that early trauma, such as abuse and/or neglect, causes changes in the activity of the HPA axis, which are seen in excessive or reduced levels of cortisols (according to Jaffee & Christian, 2014). Research also confirms that the genes that regulate the activities of the corticotropin-releasing hormone and the HPA axis show variability as a result of exposure to abuse (Tyrka et al., 2009).

On the basis of research so far, two directions of the effects of abuse and early traumatic experiences on the function of the HPA axis have been confirmed. The first presumes that in stressful situations cortisol is released without control and in excess, and its level remains high even after the effects of stress have ended, which may as a result lead to anxiety (Bremner & Vermetten, 2001; Teicher et al., 2003). Researchers who studied cortisol levels in children exposed to abuse confirmed the dysregulation of the HPA axis, which is seen in increased cortisol levels (Bruce, Fisher, Pears, & Levine, 2009; van der Vegt, van der Ende, Kirschbaum, Verhulst, & Tiemeier, 2009). The other direction of the effects of exposure to abuse on the function of the HPA axis presumes that the negative experience leads to dysfunction seen in the reduced release of cortisol. Research confirms that stress in different periods of life leads to the insufficient release of cortisol (Raison & Miller, 2003). Findings of a reduction in its levels during exposure to various stressors have also been confirmed in laboratory research. Researchers study changes in cortisol levels during the performance of various stressful tasks (e.g., public presentations), in laboratory conditions in adults with experience of abuse, and a comparable group which was not exposed to abuse (Carpenter, Shattuck, Tyrka, Geracioti, &Price, 2011; Heim et al., 2000b; MacMillan et al., 2009). Despite the different methodologies for inducing stress in laboratory conditions, the results obtained are consistent and indicate the low reactivity, that is, the weakened response of cortisol in adults with experiences of abuse in childhood (De Bellis, 2005; Heim et al., 2000a).

Many behavioural difficulties, such as aggressiveness, withdrawal, anxiety etc., are also linked to abuse and the lower reactivity of the HPA axis (Ouellet-Morin et al., 2011). In children exposed to abuse, disorders have been noticed in changes in the cortisol circadian rhythm. Particularly low cortisol levels were obtained in the morning hours (Dozier et al., 2006; Fisher, Stoolmiller, Gunnar, & Burraston, 2007; Fisher, Van Ryzin, & Gunnar, 2011) and the results of previous research (Cicchetti & Rogosch, 2001b) showed that the quantity of cortisol released also depends on the type of abuse. Higher morning levels of cortisol were evident in cases of physical and sexual abuse, whilst in children exposed only to physical forms of abuse, low levels of morning cortisol were found.

Abnormalities in the function of the HPA axis in reaction to a traumatic event also cause changes in some parts of the limbic system (Carrion et al., 2009; Choi, Jeong, Polcari, Rohan, &Teicher, 2012; De Bellis & Kuchibhatla, 2006; Tarullo & Gunnar, 2006; Tomoda, Ann, Anderson, & Teicher, 2012). The strongest changes take place in the area of the hippocampus, and include its atrophy (Tsavoussis, Stawicki, Stoicea, & Papadimos, 2014). Regarding research into the effects of abuse in childhood causing changes to different areas of the brain, the findings of relevant research will be explained in more detail below.

Traumatic experiences of abuse also affect various neurotransmitter systems, and there are increasing indications of its effect on GABA and glutamate. In normal conditions GABA inhibits the effect of glutamates, which results in reducing anxiety and the experience of stress, and contributes to the successful filtering of important and unimportant information (Wilson, Hansen, & Li, 2011). However, after a traumatic experience of abuse, the activity of the GABA neurotransmitter is reduced, which in the end reduces the possibility of separation of important and unimportant information. In children exposed to abuse in childhood reduced activity has also been found of monoamine oxidase A, the enzyme which breaks down monoamines, and this may result in a risk of depression etc. Abused persons could be at increased risk of developing autoimmune disorders (Chrosusos, 1995; Raison & Miller, 2003). In them higher levels of cytokine were found (Bertone-Johnson, Whitcomb, Missmer, Karlson, & Rich-Edwards, 2012; Kiecold-Glaser et al., 2011; Slopen, Kubzansky, McLaughlin, & Koenen, 2013), which are known to additionally activate the HPA axis in stressful situations, increasing its work. Binding itself to its receptors in the brain, excessive cytokine release impairs the glucocortiokoid hormone (Jaffee & Christian, 2014), which in the end may lead to various forms of cognitive disorders.

3. The Effect of Maltreatment in Childhood on the Function of Different Regions of the Central Nervous System

Researchers agree regarding the many changes in different parts of the central nervous system which may be linked to experience of maltreatment in childhood. Briefly, changes have been found in the frontal cortex and the limbic system, that is, in the areas included in strategic planning and decision making, processing fear and experiencing satisfaction and pleasure (Disseth, 2005; De Bellis, 2005; Heim & Nemroff, 2001; Wilson et al., 2011). It has to be said that the biological response to traumatic experiences of abuse is extremely complex due to the reciprocal and complex interactions of different parts of the nervous system. In order to simplify the presentation the key areas of the brain will be presented which change under the influence of a traumatic experience such as maltreatment in childhood.

3.1. The Limbic System

An area of the central nervous system which may be significantly affected by abuse is the limbic system, which is deemed to be the "emotional centre" of the brain. This system includes the limbic cortex (the cingulate gyrus and parahippocampal gyrus), the hippocampal formation (dentate gyrus, hippocampus and subicular complex), the amygdala, the septal area and the hypothalamus (RajMohan & Mohandas, 2007). Of these parts, the consequences of abuse are especially visible in the area of the hippocampus and the amygdala. Therefore, in this paper the emphasis will be first on the consequences of abuse on the function of these areas, and then on the remaining parts of the limbic system. The neurons of the hippocampus, which have an important role in memory and spatial orientation, are especially sensitive to stressful and traumatic events, such as maltreatment in childhood. Their heightened sensitivity is probably increased by the long period of development after birth and maturation, the presence of glucocorticoid receptors and the large-scale production of neurons which are created in this area after birth. Researches so far has connected increased quantities of glucocorticoids released in stressful situations with reduced growth of neurons in the hippocampus and with disturbances in their myleination (van der Kolk, 2003; Teicher, Anderson, & Polcari, 2012). As has already been said, atrophy of the hippocampus neurons is also linked to excessive release of cortisols. It is well-known that glucocorticoid receptors are located most densely precisely in the area of the hippocampus (Sapolsky, Krey, & NcEwen, 1986). The increased release of glucocorticoids caused by stress also causes increased production of glutamates which release the hippocampus neurons and have been connected to memory deficit (Radley & Morrison, 2005). Research confirms that prolonged stress also causes cell death and the reduced volume of the hippocampus (Harvey, Brand, Jeeva, & Stein, 2006; Shin, Rauch, & Pitman, 2006; Radley & Morrison, 2005), whilst the increased production of glutamates has been linked to structural synaptic changes to hippocampus neurons (Radley & Morrison, 2005). Many results of research to date confirm that in persons with experience of abuse in childhood the area of the white matter (which coordinates communication among the regions of the brain) and the grey matter in the hippocampus are smaller than in individuals who have not been abused (Andersen et al., 2008; Dannlowski et al., 2012; Frodl, Reinhold, Koutsouleris, Reiser, & Meisenzahl, 2010; Thomaes et al., 2010). These results, however, are not in line with the findings of two studies which took into consideration the time that had passed since the traumatic event. Bonne et al., (2011), in a sample of 37 persons aged from 18 to 65 years who were exposed to abuse, measured the volume of the hippocampus and tested the presence of post-traumatic stress symptoms, one week and six months after the traumatic event. Although the authors established the presence of post-traumatic stress disorder (PTSD) in 10 subjects, in the sample as a whole they did not find abnormalities in the volume of the hippocampus. Testing differences in the volume of the hippocampus between people with and without development of post-traumatic stress symptoms did not show any significant differences in the volume of the left and right hippocampus, one week and six months after the traumatic event. De Bellis, Hall, Boring and Moritz (2001) also had similar results when they observed the effects of abuse of children of an average age of about 10 years, immediately and two years after exposure to abuse. The authors also did not find differences in the volume of the hippocampus, and they explained the results obtained by the gradual development of the changes to the brain caused by abuse. Regarding the effects of trauma to the hippocampus neurons, the developmental period in which the abuse took place must certainly be taken into account. Some studies (De Bellis et al., 2001; Teicher et al., 2003) confirm the importance of the sex, but also the age of the children. Since neurogenesis in the area of the hippocampus begins post-conception, abnormalities in the size of the hippocampus may be visible even before puberty, when the peak of neurogenesis and synaptic bonding occurs. However, De Bellis et al., (2001) state that the consequences of abuse are not necessarily visible in that period because neurogenesis masks the present loss of neurons and thereby reduces the possibility of changes to the hippocampus caused by the stress and trauma of abuse. It has been confirmed that the changes are more visible in boys than in girls, because the process of neurogenesis, primarily the myelination processes, occurs earlier in boys than in girls (Teicher et al., 2003). As was said earlier, the consequences of abuse are also visible in the function of the amygdala, the main part of the limbic system. The amygdala is important in regulating various emotions, and it has a key role in recognizing, conditioning and expressing fear (Olsson & Phelps, 2007). This part of the limbic system functions as a "danger detector". It is mainly influenced by the system of vision, but also other sensor modalities, and the amygdala evaluates potentially threatening stimuli from the environment. When danger is detected, the amygdala sends its response to other parts of the nervous system (e.g., the hypothalmus), which in the end leads to a "fight or flight" reaction. In connections with the hippocampus, the amygdala has an important role in assessing the emotional value of the stimulus (Phelps, 2004) and takes control of behaviour, even while the prefrontal cortex is still in the phase of processing a suitable reaction. Remembering trauma may cause the activation of the amygdala, an inappropriate "fight or flight" reaction, or even a "freeze" reaction. Exaggerated reactions to stimuli related to trauma increase the level of arousal of the organism and prevent learning from experience (Cohen, Perel, De Bellis, Friedman, &Putnam, 2002; Shin et al., 2006). The very activation of the amygdala activates the neuroendocrine system, which results in the heightened secretion of cortisol and adrenalin, which prepare the organism for a behaviour response. The final reaction resembles dissociative symptoms, excluding an emotional response, with limited awareness of external events and reduced concentration (Disseth, 2005).

The findings of recent research show that in abused and neglected children, in comparison with a control group of children, the amygdala had greater volume (Mehta et al., 2009; Tottenham et al., 2010), and there is greater basal activity in the area of the amygdala nuclei (McCrory et al., 2013; Woon & Hedges, 2009). The increased activity of the amygdala is expressed in performing tasks which include recognizing the emotional expressions of anger and happiness. In children exposed to abuse research also confirms the increased activation of the right amygdala in recognizing anger in relation to neutral faces (McCrory et al., 2013).

Other areas of the limbic system which react to abuse as a stressful traumatic event mentioned in the literature are the cingulate cortex and the nucleus of the basal ganglia. For example, in some studies cerebral blood flow was tested, measured using positron emission tomography, in women who were victims of sexual abuse in childhood, and who developed PTSD (Bremner et al., 1999). The women listened to stories with traumatic content, and while this task was being performed their cerebral blood flow was measured. The results obtained showed an increase in blood flow in the regions of the prefrontal cortex, the hippocampus and the hypothalamus, which are included in the traumatic stress response. Other studies also report an increase in blood flow in the visually association cortex, the motor cortex and the cingulate cortex in women who had experienced PTSD (Wilson et al., 2011). The cingulate cortex has many connections with the amygdala and other parts of the limbic system and neocortex, and its function is to transfer forms of reaction or decisions related to stimuli. In other words, the cingulate cortex detects conflict and "mistakes" and proposes the most desirable actions (Magno, Foxe, Molholm, Robertson, & Garavan, 2006), which are not always appropriate. In people exposed to abuse, this reaction by the cingulate cortex is often mistaken because it is based on a mistaken interpretation of all events as threatening, which creates a basis for a maladaptive strategies in reactions. Research also reports the reduced size of the anterior cingulate cortex and the caudal nucleus in abused persons (Andersen & Teicher, 2004; van

Goozen et al., 2007). The neural path based on incorrect or inadequate assessment of an event in a person exposed to abuse may begin on the level of the thalamus, which passes information on to the amygdala and the cingulate cortex (Wilson et al., 2011). Since making decisions about how to react and the very experience of a stressful situation begins on the level of the thalamus, researchers were interested in whether there is a difference in the volume of this subcortical nucleus between abused and non-abused persons. Research reports the increased activity of the locus coeruleus nucleus, accompanied by increased adrenalin activity, in children who were traumatized in childhood (Wilson et al., 2011). These results could also have been expected, taking into account the fact that the locus coeruleus is the major noradrenergic nucleus (Vermetten & Bremner, 2002a, 2002b) and that in threatening situations it induces the excessive production of catecholamine (Wilson et al., 2011), which in the end prevents the function of the cortical areas that are important for adequate control of reactions. On the basis of the results of research so far, it may be concluded that in abused persons there is increased activity in the limbic system, or some of its parts, which certainly contributes to imbalance and decreased activity in the prefrontal cortex.

3.2. The Prefrontal Cortex

The prefrontal cortex regulates understanding, planning, judgement, verbal skills and working memory (Weber & Reynolds, 2004). Its role is also important in the regulation and maintenance of attention, and in selection of important and less important information (Weber & Reynolds, 2004). The prefrontal cortex develops up until the early 20's, when it achieves its full volume, thanks to the processes of maturation and myelination. Since its function is formed gradually, the effects of early negative experience are only possible in later periods in life, when this part of the cortex reaches its functional and/or structural maturity. Recent studies confirm the reduced area of the frontal lobe, and the reduced functions related to control of behaviour, changes of personality, and control of movement and other executive functions, in persons exposed to maltreatment (Richert, Carrion, Karchemshkiy, & Reiss, 2006; Shin et al., 2006; Teicher, Samson, Tomoda, Ashy, & Andersen, 2006). Richert et al., (2006), using magnetic resonance, tested the consequences of post-traumatic experience on the function of the frontal lobe in a sample of children aged from 7 to 14 years, of whom most had developed PTSD as a result of witnessing family violence (40%), physical violence (37%), sexual abuse (20%), physical neglect (12%), and emotional abuse (7%), multiple maltreatment (55%), or separation and loss (55%). The study included a comparable (control) group of children who had not been exposed to traumatic experiences. The results showed differences in the volume of the prefrontal grey matter between the groups. Children exposed to a traumatic experience had a smaller prefrontal cortex in comparison with the control group, whilst in the other areas of the brain (the middle and anterior areas) the volume increased. Research so far also confirms that adolescence is the most sensitive period, in terms of changes to the prefrontal cortex caused by the trauma of abuse (Teicher, 2005).

3.3. The Corpus Callosum

The corpus callosum, which links the left and right cerebral hemispheres, shows changes due to exposure to maltreatment in childhood. It has been shown that high levels of glucocorticoids interfere with the myelination of its axons during development, preventing the creation of myelin, which results in the slower transfer of nerve impulses between the two hemispheres of the brain (Teicher et al., 2003). Findings to date confirm that maltreatment in childhood has a negative effect on the development of the corpus callosum (Cohen et al., 2002; Teicher et al., 2004, 2006), and this depends on the sex and the type of abuse and neglect to which the child was exposed. In boys the reduction in size of the corpus callosum is linked to neglect, and in girls the strongest negative effect on the size of the corpus callosum results from sexual abuse (Teicher et al., 2003).

Exposure to maltreatment in childhood also affects the development of the left hemisphere, and this finding is supported by the results of neurophysiological tests. Teicher (2000) compared the results of two groups of people who suffer from mental illnesses, of which one group had experience of maltreatment in childhood, whilst the other group had not been abused. The author compared the results they found in tests of visual-spatial skills (for which the right hemisphere is dominant), and verbal skills (dominant left hemisphere). In the group which was not abused, deficits in tests linked to the function of the left hemisphere were twice as frequent in comparison with deficits related to functions of the right hemisphere. However, in persons exposed to physical, sexual or psychological abuse, deficits of the left hemisphere were six times more expressed than deficits of the right hemisphere. The greatest deficits in the function of the left hemisphere were visible in persons exposed to psychological abuse (up to eight times). In addition, Teicher et al., (2003) established that abused individuals use the right hemisphere more when remembering disturbing events, and the left hemisphere when remembering neutral events. In this research the control group of participants activated both hemispheres equally when remembering disturbing and neutral events.

CONCLUSION

On the basis of a review of research undertaken to date it is possible to offer a fairly simple perception of the various neurobiological changes that take place in persons exposed to maltreatment in childhood. The changes documented by research so far are evident in the neuroendocrine systems activated by stress (the sympathetic nervous system and the HPA axis) and in various regions of the limbic system (especially the hippocampus and the amygdala), and the prefrontal cortex. The development of the corpus callosum is also affected by abuse as a traumatic event. From the results of the research so far it follows that when studying the mechanisms by which abuse affects various neurobiological systems, factors must not be overlooked such as the age at which the abuse took place, the child's sex, and the severity and form of abuse to which the child was exposed. These factors individually, and their interactive effect, may change the mechanisms of the effect of abuse on neurobiological processes. It is difficult to establish a pure and clear connection between maltreatment in childhood and various neural changes because many individuals and environmental factors may have a mediating role in the relationship between traumatic experiences and neurobiological development. Also, when drawing conclusions on the consequences of maltreatment in childhood it is necessary to take into account the differences in methodologies of research which are reflected in the different samples of participants in the research, and in the use of different techniques and measurement instruments.

REFERENCES

Andersen, S. L., & Teicher M. H. (2004). Delayed effects of early stress on hippocampal development. *Neuropsychopharmacology*, 29(11), 1988-1993. doi: 10.1038/sj.npp.1300528.

Andersen, S. L., Tomada, A., Vincow, E. S., Valente, E., Polcari, A., & Teicher, M. H. (2008). Preliminary evidence for sensitive periods in the effect of childhood sexual abuse on regional brain development. *Journal of Neuropsychiatry and Clinical Neurosciences*, 20(3), 292-301.doi: 10.1176/jnp.2008.20.3.292.

Bertone-Johnson, E. R., Whitcomb, B. W., Missmer, S. A., Karlson, E. W., & Rich-Edwards, J. W. (2012). Inflammation and early-life abuse in women. *American Journal of Preventive Medicine*, 43(6), 611-620. doi: 10.1016/j.amepre.2012.08.014.

Bonne, O., Brandes, D., Gilboa, A., Gomori, J. M., Shenton, M. E., Pitman, R. K., & Shaley, A. Y. (2001). Longitudinal MRI study of hippocampal volume in trauma survivors with PTSD. *The American Journal of Psychiatry*, 158(8), 1248-1251. doi:10.1176/ appi.ajp.158.8.1248.

Bremner, J. D. (2006). Traumatic stress: effects on the brain. *Dialogues in Clinical Neuroscience*, 8(4), 445-461.

Bremner, J. D., Narayan, M., Staib, L. H., Southwick, S. M., McGlashan, T., & Charney, D. S. (1999). Neural correlates of memories of childhood sexual abuse in women with and without posttraumatic stress disorder. *The American Journal of Psychiatry*, 156(11), 1787-1795. doi: 10.1176/ajp.156.11.1787.

Bremner, J. D., & Vermetten, E. (2001). Stress and development: Behavioral and biological consequences. *Development and Psychopathology*, 13(3), 473-489.

Bromfield, L., &Higgins, D. (2005). National comparison of child protection systems: Child Abuse Prevention Issues. *Australian Institute of Family Studies*, 22. Retrieved from www.aifs.gov.au/nch/pubs/issues/issues22/issues22.html.

Bruce, J., Fisher, P. A., Pears, K. C., & Levine, S. (2009). Morning cortisol levels in preschool-aged foster children: Differential effects of maltreatment type. *Developmental Psychobiology*, 51(1), 14-23. doi:10.1002/dev.20333.

Bryant, R. A., Harvey, A. G., Gurhtie, R. M., & Moulds, M. L.(2000). A prospective study of psychophysiological arousal, acute stress disorder and posttraumtic stress disorder. *Journal of Abnormal Psychology*, 109(2), 341-344. doi: 10.1037/0021-843X.109.2.341.

Carpenter, L. L., Shattuck, T. T., Tyrka, A. R., Geracioti, T. D., &Price, L. H. (2011). Effect of childhood physical abuse on cortisol stress response. *Psychopharmacology*, 214(1), 367-375. doi:10.1007/s00213-010-2007-4.

Carrion, V. G., Weems, C. F., Watson, C., Eliez, S., Menon, V., &Reiss, A. L. (2009). Converging evidence for abnormalities of the prefrontal cortex and evaluation of midsagittal structures in pediatric posttraumatic stress disorder: an MRI study. *Psychiatry Resesearch*, 172(3), 226-234. doi: 10.1016/j.pscychresns.2008.07.008.

Casey, B. J., Giedd, J. N., &Thomas, K. M. (2000). Structural and functional brain development and its relation to cognitive development. *Biological Psychiatry*, 54(1-3), 241-257. doi: 10.1016/S0301-0511(00)00058-2.

Choi, J., Jeong, B., Polcari, A., Rohan, M. L., &Teicher, M. H. (2012). Reduced fractional anisotropy in the visual limbic pathway of young adults witnessing domestic violence in childhood. *Neuroimage*, 59(2), 1071-1079. doi: 10.1016/j.neuroimage.2011.09.033.

Cicchetti, D., &Rogosch, F. A. (2001b). Diverse patterns of neuroendocrine activity in maltreated children. *Development and Psychopathology*, 13(3), 677-693. doi: 10.1017/S0954579401003145.

Cohen, J. A., Perel, J. M., De Bellis, M. D., Friedman, M. J., &Putnam, F. W. (2002). Treating traumatizes children, clinical implications of the psychobiology of posttraumatic stress disorder. *Trauma, Violence, & Abuse*, 3(2), 91-108. doi: 10.1177/15248380020032001.

Cook, F., Ciorciari, J., Varker, T., & Devilly, G. J. (2009). Changes in long term neural connectivity following psychological trauma. *Clinical Neurophysiology*, 120(2), 309-314. doi: 10.1016/j.clinph.2008.11.021.

Cornwall, M. (2016). *Go suck a lemon: Strategies for improving your emotional intelligence*. Charleston: Createspace Independent.

Dannlowski, U., Stuhrmann, A., Beutelmann, V., Zwanzger, P., Lenzen, T., Grotegerd, D., Domschke, K., Hohoff, C., Ohrmann, P., Bauer, J., Lindner, C., Postert, C., Konrad, C., Arolt, V., Heindel, W., Suslow, T., & Kugel, H. (2012). Limbic scars: Long-term consequences of childhood maltreatment revealed by functional and structural magnetic resonance imaging. *Biological Psychiatry*, 71(4), 286-293. doi: 10.1016/j.biopsych.2011.10.021.

De Bellis, M. D. (2005). The psychobiology of neglect. *Child Maltreatment*, 10(2), 150-172. doi: 10.1177/1077559505275116.

De Bellis, M. D. (2007). Developmental traumatology: a contributory mechanism for alcohol and substance use disorders. *Psychoneuroendocrinology*, 27(1-2), 155-170. doi: 10.1016/S0306-4530(01)00042-7.

De Bellis, M. D., Hall, J., Boring, A. M., Frustaci, K., & Moritz, G. (2001). A pilot longitudinal study of hippocampal volume in pediatric maltreated-related posttraumatic stress disorder. *Society of Biological Psychiatry*, 50(4), 305-309. doi:10.1016/S0006-3223(01)01105-2.

De Bellis, M. D., Keshavan, M. S., Clark, D. B., Casey, B. J., Giedd, J. N., Boring, A. M., Frustaci, K., & Ryan, N. D. (1999). Developmental traumatology part II: Brain development. *Biological Psychiatry*, 45(10), 1271-1284. doi: 10.1016/S0006-3223(99)00045-1.

De Bellis, M. D., Keshavan, M. S., Shifflett, H., Iyengar, S., Beers, S. R., Hall, J., & Moritz, G. (2002). Brain structures in pediatric maltreatment-related posttraumatic stress disorder: A sociodemographically matched study. *Biological Psychiatry*, 52(11), 1066-1078. doi:10.1016/S0006-3223(02)01459-2.

De Bellis, M. D., & Kuchibhatla, M. (2006). Cerebellar volumes in pediatric maltreatment-related posttraumatic stress disorder. *Biological Psychiatry*, 60(7), 697-703. doi: 10.1016/j.biopsych.2006.04.035.

Delima, J., &Vimpani, G. (2011). The neurobiological effects of childhood maltreatment: an often overlooked narrative related to the long-term effects of early childhood trauma? *Family Matters*, 89, 42-52.

Disseth, T. H. (2005). Dissociation in children and adolescents as reaction to trauma- on overview of conceptual issues and neurobiological factors. *Nordic Journal of Psychiatry*, 59(2), 79-91. doi: 10.1080/08039480510022963.

Dozier, M., Manni, M., Gordon, M. K., Peloso, E., Gunnar, M. R., Stovall-McClough, K. C., Eldreth, D., & Levine, S. (2006). Foster children's diurnal production of cortisol: An exploratory study. *Child Maltreatment*, 11(2), 189-197. doi: 10.1177/1077559505285779.

Durston, S., Hulshoff, P., Hilleke, E., Casey, B. J., Giedd, J. N., Buitelaar, J. K., & van Engeland, H. (2001). Anatomical MRI of the developing human brain: what have we learned? *Journal of the American Academy of Child and Adolescent Psychiatry*, 40(9), 1012-1020. doi: 10.1097/00004583-200109000-00009.

Ethier, L., Lemelin, J. P., & Lacharite, C. (2004). A longitudinal study of the effects of chronic maltreatment on children's behavioral and emotional problems. *Child Abuse & Neglect*, 28(12), 1265-1278. doi: 10.1016/j.chiabu.2004.07.006.

Finkelhor, D., Ormrod, R. K., Turner, H. A., & Hamby, S. L. (2005). Measuring poly-victimization using the Juvenile Victimization Questionnaire. *Child Abuse & Neglect*, 29(11), 1297-1312. doi: 10.1016/j.chiabu.2005.06.005.

Fisher, P. A., Stoolmiller, M., Gunnar, M. R., & Burraston, B. O. (2007). Effects of a therapeutic intervention for foster preschoolers on diurnal cortisol activity. *Psychoneuroendocrinology*, 32(8-10), 892-905. doi: 10.1016/j.psyneuen.2007.06.008.

Fisher, P. A., Van Ryzin, M. J., & Gunnar, M. R. (2011). Mitigating HPA axis dysregulation associated with placement changes in foster care. *Psychoneuroendocrinology*, 36(4), 531-539. doi: 10.1016/ j.psyneuen.2010.08.007.

French, W. P. (2008). Neurobiology of violence and victimization. In T. W. Miller (Ed.), *School violence and primary prevention* (pp. 25-58). New York: Springer.

Frodl, T., Reinhold, E., Koutsouleris, N., Reiser, M., & Meisenzahl, E. M. (2010). Interaction of childhood stress with hippocampus and prefrontal cortex volume reduction in major depression. *Journal of Psychiatric Research*, 44(13), 799-807. doi: 10.1016/j.jpsychires. 2010.01.006.

Giedd, J. N., Blumenthal, J., & Jeffries, N. O. (1999). Development of the normal human corpus callosum during childhood and adolescence: a longitudinal MRI study. *Progress in Neuropsychopharmacology and Biological Psychiatry*, 23(4), 571-588. doi: 10.1016/S0278-5846(99)00017-2.

Giedd, J. N., Blumenthal, J., Jeffries, N. O., Castellanos, F. X., Liu, H., Zijdenbos, A., Paus, T., Evans, A. C., & Rapoport, J. L. (1999). Brain development during childhood and adolescence: a longitudinal MRI study. *Nature Neuroscience*, 2, 861-863.doi:10.1038/13158.

Giedd, J. N., Castellanos, F. X., Rajapakse, J. C., Vaituzis, A. C, & Rapoport, J. L. (1997). Sexual dimorphism of the developing human brain. *Progress in Neuropsychopharmacology and Biological Psychiatry*, 21(8), 1185-1201. doi: 10.1016/S0278-5846(97)00158-9.

Giedd, J. N., Snell, J. W., Lange, N., Rajapakse, J. C., Casey, B. J., Kozuch, P. L., Vaituzis, A. C., Vauss, Y. C., Hamburger, S. D., Kaysen, D., & Rapoport, J. L. (1996a). Quantitative magnetic resonance imaging of human brain development:Ages 14-18. *Cerebral Cortex*, 6(4), 551-560.

Giedd, J. N., Vaituzis, A. C., Hamburger, S. D., Lange, N., Rajapakse, J. C., Kaysen, D., Vauss, Y. C., Rapoport, J. L. (1996b): Quantitative MRI of the temporal lobe, amygdala, and hippocampus in normal human development: ages 4-18 years. *Journal of Comparative Neurology*, 366, 223-230.

Graham, J. C., English, D. J., Litrownik, A. J., Thompson, R., Briggs, E. C., & Bangdiwala, S. I. (2010). Maltreatment chronicity defined with reference to development: Extension of the social adaptation outcomes findings to peer relations. *Journal of Family Violence*, 25(3), 311-324. doi: 10.1007/s10896-009-9293-9.

Harvey, B. H., Brand, L., Jeeva, Z., & Stein, D. J. (2006). Cortical/hippocampal monoamines, HPA-axis changes and aversive behavior following stress and restress in an animal model of post-traumatic stress disorder. *Physiology and Behavior*, 87(5), 881-890. doi: 10.1016/j.physbeh.2006.01.033.

Heim, C., Ehlert, U., & Hellhammer, D. H. (2000a). The potential role of hypocortisolism in the pathophysiology of stress-related bodily disorders. *Psychoneuroendocrinology*, 25(1), 1-35. doi: 10.1016/S0306-4530(99)00035-9.

Heim, C., & Nemeroff, C. B. (2001). The role of childhood trauma in the neurobiology of mood and anxiety disorders: preclinical and clinical studies. *Biological Psychiatry*, 49(12), 1023-1039. doi: 10.1016/S0006-3223(01)01157-X.

Heim, C., Newport, D. J., Heit, S., Graham, Y. P., Wilcox, M., Bonsall, R., & Nemeroff, C.B. (2000b). Pituitary-adrenal and autonomic responses to stress in women after sexual and physical abuse in childhood.

Journal of the American Medical Association, 284(5), 592-597. doi: :10.1001/jama.284.5.592.

Higgins, D., & McCabe, M. (2001). Multiple forms of child abuse and neglect: Adult retrospective reports. *Aggression and Violent Behaviour*, 6(6), 547-578. doi: 10.1016/S1359-1789(00)00030-6.

Jaffee, S. R., & Christian, C. W. (2014). The biological embedding of child abuse and neglect implications for policy and practice. *Social Policy Report*, 28(1), 1-36.

Jernigan, T. L., Archibald, S. L., Berhow, M. T., Sowell, E. R., Foster, D. S., & Hesselink, J. R. (1991). Cerebral structure on MRI, Part I: Localization of age-related changes. *Biological Psychiatry*, 29(1), 55-67. doi: 10.1016/0006-3223(91)90210-D.

Kiecolt-Glaser, J. K., Gouin, J. P., Weng, N. P., Malarkey, W. B., Beversdorf, D. Q., & Glaser, R. (2011). Childhood adversity heightens the impact of later-life caregiving stress on telomere length and inflammation. *Psychosomatic Medicine*, 73(1), 16-22. doi: 10.1097/PSY.0b013e31820573b6.

Kitzmann, K.M., Gaylord, N. K., Holt, A. R., & Kenny, E. D. (2003). Child witnesses to domestic violence: a meta-analytic review. *Journal of Consulting and Clinical Psychology*, 71(2), 339-352. doi: 10.1037/0022-006X.71.2.339.

Levendosky, A. A., Bogat, G. A., & Martinez-Torteya, C. (2013). PTSD symptoms in young children exposed to intimate partner violence. *Violence Against Women*, 19(2), 187-201. doi: 10.1177/1077801213476458.

Lorenz, T. K., Harte, C.B., & Meston, C. M. (2015). Changes in autonomic nervous system activity are associated with changes in sexual function in women with a history of childhood sexual abuse. *Journal of Sexual Medicine*, 12(7), 1545-1554. doi: 10.1111/jsm.12908.

MacMillan, H. L., Georgiades, K., Duku, E. K., Shea, A., Steiner, M., Niec, A., Tanaka, M., Gensey, S., Spree, S., Vella, E., Walsh, C. A., De Bellis, M. D., van der Meulen, J., Boyle, M. H., & Schmidt, L. A. (2009). Cortisol response to stress in female youths exposed to childhood maltreatment: Results of the Youth Mood Project.

Biological Psychiatry, 66 (1), 62-68. doi: 10.1016/j.biopsych. 2008.12.014.

Magno, E., Foxe, J. J., Molholm, S., Robertson, I. H., & Garavan, H. (2006). The anterior cingulate and error avoidance. *Journal of Neuroscience*, 26(18), 4769-4773. doi: 10.1523/JNEUROSCI.0369-06.2006.

McCrory, E. J., De Brito, S. A., Kelly, P. A., Bird, G., Sebastian, C. L., Mechelli, A., Samuel, S., & Viding, E. (2013). Amygdala activation in maltreated children during pre-attentive emotional processing. *British Journal of Psychiatry*, 202(4), 269-276. doi: 10.1192/ bjp.bp.112.116624.

Mehta, M. A., Golembo, N. I., Nosarti, C., Colvert, E., Mota, A., Williams, S. C., Rutter, M., & Sonuga-Barke, E. J. (2009). Amygdala, hippocampal and corpus callosum size following severe early institutional deprivation: The English and Romanian Adoptees Study Pilot. *Journal of Child Psychology and Psychiatry*, 50(8), 943-951. doi: 10.1111/j.1469-7610.2009.02084.x.

Miller-Perrin, C., & Perrin, R. (2007). *Child maltreatment: An introduction*. Thousand Oaks: Sage Publications.

Murray-Close, D., Holland, A. S., & Roisman, G. I. (2012). Autonomic arousal and relational aggression in heterosexual dating couples. *Personal Relationships*, 19(2), 203-18. doi: 10.1111/j.1475-6811.2011.01348.x.

Olsson, A., & Phelps, E. A. (2007). Social learning of fear. *Nature Neuroscience*, 10, 1095-1102. doi: 10.1038/nn1968.

Ouellet-Morin, I., Odgers, C. L., Danese, A., Bowes, L., Shakoor, S., Papadopoulos, A. S., Caspi, A., Moffitt, T. E., & Arseneault, L. (2011). Blunted cortisol responses to stress signal social and behavioral problems among maltreated/bullied 12-year-old children. *Biological Psychiatry*, 70(11), 1016-1023. doi: 10.1016/ j.biopsych.2011.06.017.

Paus, T., Zijdenbos, A., Worsley, K., Collins, D. L., Blumenthal, J., Giedd, J. N., Rapoport, J. L., & Evans, A. C. (1999). Structural maturation of neural pathways in children and adolescents: *In vivo* study. *Science*, 283(5409), 1908-1911. doi: 10.1126/science.283.5409.1908.

Pfefferbaum, A., Mathalon, D. H., Sullivan, E. V., Rawles, J. M., Zipursky, R. B., & Lim, K. O. (1994). A quantitative magnetic resonance imaging study of changes in brain morphology from infancy to late adulthood. *Archives of Neurology*, 51(9), 874-887. doi: 10.1001/archneur.1994.00540210046012.

Phelps, E. A. (2004). Human emotion and memory: Interactions of the amygdala and hippocampal complex. *Current Opinion in Neurobiology*, 14(2), 198-202. doi: 10.1016/j.conb.2004.03.015.

Porges, S. W. (2009). Stress and Parasympathetic Control. In L.R Squire (Ed), *Encyclopedia of neuroscience* (pp. 463-469). Oxford: Academic Press.

Price-Robertson, R., Rush, P., Wall, L., & Higgins, D. (2013). Rarely an isolated incident: Acknowledging the interrelatedness of child maltreatment, victimisation and trauma. *Child Family Community Australia*, 15. Retrieved from https://aifs.gov.au/cfca/publications/ effects-child-abuse-and-neglect-children-and-adolescents.

Radley, J., & Morrison, J. (2005). Repeated stress and structural plasticity in the brain. *Ageing Research Reviews*, 4(2), 271-287. doi: 10.1016/j.arr.2005.03.004.

Raison, C. L., & Miller, A. H. (2003). When not enough is too much: The role of insufficient glucocorticoid signaling in the pathophysiology of stress-related disorders. *American Journal of Psychiatry*, 160(9), 1554-1565. doi: 10.1176/appi.ajp.160.9.1554.

RajMohan, V., & Mohandas E. (2007). The limbic system. *Indian Journal of Psychiatry*, 49(2), 132-139. doi: 10.4103/0019-5545.33264.

Rapoport, J. L., Giedd, J. N., Blumenthal, J., Hamburger, S., Jeffries, N., Fernandez, T., Nicolson, R., Bedwell, J., Lenane, M., Zijdenbos, A., Paus, T., & Evans, A. (1999). Progressive cortical change during adolescence in childhood-onset schizophrenia: A longitudinal magnetic resonance imaging study. *Archives of General Psychiatry*, 56(7), 649-654. doi: 10.1001/archpsyc.56.7.649.

Richert, K. A., Carrion, V. G., Karchemshkiy, A., & Reiss, A. L. (2006). Regional difference of the prefrontal cortex in pediatric PTSD: An MRI study. *Depression and Anxiety*, 23(1), 17-25. doi: 10.1002/da.20131.

Sapolsky, R. M., Krey, L. C., & McEwen, B. S. (1986). The neuroendocrinology of stress and aging: The glucocorticoid cascade hypothesis. *Endocrine Reviews*, 7(3), 284-301. doi: 10.1210/edrv-7-3-284.

Shin, L. M., Rauch, S. L., & Pitman, R. K. (2006). Amygdala, medial prefrontal cortex, and hippocampal function in PTSD. *Annals of the New York Academy of Sciences*, 1071, 67-97. doi: 10.1196/annals.1364.007.

Slopen, N., Kubzansky, L. D., McLaughlin, K. A., & Koenen, K. C. (2013). Childhood adversity and inflammatory processes in youth: A prospective study. *Psychoneuroendocrinology*, 38(2), 188-200. doi: 10.1016/j.psyneuen.2012.05.013.

Sowell, E. R., Thompson, P. M., Holmes, C. J., Batth, R., Jernigan, T. L., & Toga, A. W. (1999). Localizing age-related changes in brain structure between childhood and adolescence using statistical parametric mapping. *Neuroimage*, 9(6), 587-597. doi: 10.1006/nimg.1999.0436.

Streeck-Fischer, A., & van der Kolk, B. A. (2000). Down will come baby, cradle and all: Diagnostic and therapeutic implications of chronic trauma on child development. *Australian and New Zealand Journal of Psychiatry*, 34(6), 903-918. doi: 10.1080/000486700265.

Sullivan, E. V., Marsh, L., Mathalon, D. H., Lim, K. O., & Pfefferbaum, A. (1995). Age-related decline in MRI volumes of temporal gray matter but not hippocampus. *Neurobiology Aging*, 16(4), 591-606. doi: 10.1016/0197-4580(95)00074-O.

Tarullo, A. R., & Gunnar, M. R. (2006). Child maltreatment and the developing HPA axis. *Hormones and Behavior*, 50(4), 632-639. doi: 10.1016/j.yhbeh.2006.06.010.

Teicher, M. H. (2005, May). *Childhood abuse and regional brain development: Evidence for sensitive period.* Paper presented at the

69th Annual Scientific Meeting of the Society of Biological Psychiatry, New York. New York: EasyBib Publishing.

Teicher, M. H. (2000). Wounds that time won't heal: the neurobiology of child abuse. *Cerebrum*, 2(4), 50-67.

Teicher, M. H., Andersen, S. L., Polcari, A., Andersen, C. M., Navalta, C. P., & Kim, D. M. (2003). The neurobiological consequences of early stress and childhood maltreatment. *Neuroscience and Biobehavioral Reviews*, 27(1-2), 33-44. doi: 10.1016/S0149-7634(03)00007-1.

Teicher, M. H., Anderson, C. M., & Polcari, A. (2012). Childhood maltreatment is associated with reduced volume in the hippocampal subfields CA3, dentate gyrus and subiculum. *Proceedings of the National Academy of Sciences*, 109(9), 563-572. doi: 10.1073/pnas.1115396109.

Teicher, M. H., Dumont, N. L., Ito, Y., Vaituzis, C., Giedd, J. N., & Andersen, S. L. (2004). Child neglect is associated with reduced corpus callosum area. *Biological Psychiatry*, 56(2), 80-85. doi: 10.1016/j.biopsych.2004.03.016.

Teicher, M. H., Samson A., Tomoda, A., Ashy, M., & Andersen, S. L. (2006). Neurobiological and behavioral consequences of exposure to childhood traumatic stress. In B. Arnetz, & R. Ekman (Eds.), *Stress in health and disease* (pp.180-195). Germany: Wiley-VCH.

Thomaes, K., Dorrepaal, E., Draijer, N., de Ruiter, M. B., van Balkom, A. J., Smit, J. H., & Veltman, D. J. (2010). Reduced anterior cingulate and orbitofrontal volumes in child abuse-related complex PTSD. *Journal of Clinical Psychiatry*, 71(12), 1636-1644. doi: 10.4088/JCP.08m04754blu.

Thompson, P. M., Giedd, J. N., Woods, R. P., MacDonald, D., Evans, A. C., & Toga, A. W. (2000). Growth patterns in the developing brain detected by using continuum mechanical tensor maps. *Nature*, 404(6774), 190-193. doi: 10.1038/35004593.

Tomoda, A., Ann, P., Anderson, C. M., & Teicher, M. H. (2012). Reduced visual cortex gray matter volume and thickness in young adults who witnessed domestic violence during childhood. *PLoS One*, 7(12), e52528. doi: 10.1371/journal.pone.0052528.

Tottenham, N., Hare, T. A., Quinn, B. T., McCarry, T. W., Nurse, M., Gilhooly, T., Millner, A., Galvan, A., Davidson, M. C., Ejasti, I. M., Thomas, K. M., Freed, P. J., Booma, E. S., Gunnar, M. R., Alternus, M., Aronson, J., & Casey, B. J. (2010). Prolonged institutional rearing is associated with atypically large amygdala volume and difficulties in emotion regulation. *Developmental Science*, 13(1), 46-61. doi: 10.1111/j.1467-7687.2009.00852.x.

Tsavoussis, A., Stawicki, S. P. A., Stoicea, N., & Papadimos, T. J. (2014). Child-witnessed domestic violence and its adverse effects on brain development: A call for societal self-examination and awareness. *Fronteries in Public Health*, 2, 178. doi: 10.3389/fpubh.2014.00178.

Tyrka, A. R., Price, L. H., Gelernter, J., Schepker, C., Anderson, G. M., & Carpenter, L. L. (2009). Interaction of childhood maltreatment with the corticotropin-releasing hormone receptor gene: Effects on HPA axis reactivity. *Biological Psychiatry*, 66(7), 681-685. doi: 10.1016/j.biopsych.2009.05.012.

van der Kolk, A. B. (2003). The neurobiology of childhood trauma and abuse. *Child and Adolescent Psychiatric Clinics*, 12(2), 293-317. doi: 10.1016/S1056-4993(03)00003-8.

van der Vegt, E. J., van der Ende, J., Kirschbaum, C., Verhulst, F. C., & Tiemeier, H. (2009). Early neglect and abuse predict diurnal cortisol patterns in adults: A study of international adoptees. *Psychoneuroendocrinology*, 34(5), 660-669. doi: 10.1016/j.psyneuen.2008.11.004.

van Goozen, S. H. M., Fairchild, G., Snoek, H., & Harold, G. (2007). The evidence for a neurobiological model of childhood antisocial behavior. *Psychological Bulletin*, 133(1), 149-182. doi:10.1037/0033-2909.133.1.149.

Vermetten, E., & Bremner, J. D. (2002a). Circuits and systems in stress. I. Preclinical studies. *Depression and Anxiety*, 15(3), 126-147. doi: 10.1002/da.10016.

Vermetten, E., & Bremner, J. D. (2002b). Circuits and systems in stress. II. Applications to neurobiology and treatment in posttraumatic stress disorder. *Depression and Anxiety*, 16(1), 14-38. doi: 10.1002/da.10017.

Weber, D. A., & Reynolds, C. R. (2004). Clinical perspectives on neurobiological effects of psychological trauma. *Neuropsychology Review*, 14(2), 115-129. doi: 10.1023/B:NERV.0000028082.13778.14.

Wilson, K. R., Hansen, D. J., & Li, M. (2011). The traumatic stress response in child maltreatment and resultant neuropsychological effects. *Aggression and Violent Behavior*, 16(2), 87-97. doi: 10.1016/j.avb.2010.12.007.

Woon, F. L., & Hedges, D. W. (2009). Amygdala volume in adults with posttraumatic stress disorder: a meta-analysis. *Neuropsychiatry and Clinical Neurosciences*, 21(1), 5-12. doi: 10.1176/appi.neuropsych.21.1.5.

World Health Organization (2002). *World Report on Violence and Health: Summary*. Geneva: World Health Organization.

In: Horizons in Neuroscience Research ISBN: 978-1-53613-286-1
Editors: A. Costa and E. Villalba

Chapter 4

BIOMECHANICS OF THE TIBIAL NERVE: NORMAL AND PATHOLOGICAL STATES AS MEASURED BY ULTRASOUND

Anabela G. Silva*[1,2,*]*, PhD and Milton Santos*[1,3]*, PhD

[1]School of Health Sciences, University of Aveiro,
Campus Universitário de Santiago, Aveiro, Portugal
[2]CINTESIS.UA, University of Aveiro,
Campus Universitário de Santiago, Aveiro, Portugal
[3]IEETA, University of Aveiro,
Campus Universitário de Santiago, Aveiro, Portugal

ABSTRACT

Nerves in general and the tibial nerve in particular are able to respond to movement and sustained postures while maintaining their normal function. They adapt to these stresses through a variety of mechanisms, such as gliding in relation to adjacent structures, increased strain and ability to tolerate compression. These mechanisms are named nerve biomechanics. Nevertheless, it is believed that nerve biomechanics

[*] Corresponding Author Email: asilva@ua.pt.

is impaired in the presence of pathology and some health professionals, such as physiotherapists, make an attempt to restore it as a means to restore normal nerve function. However, for a comprehensive understanding of the normal tibial nerve biomechanics and how it is affected by pathology there is a need to i) characterize normal tibial nerve biomechanics, ii) changes in tibial nerve biomechanics in the presence of pathology and iii) whether these changes relate to changes in the tibial nerve function. Furthermore, nerve biomechanics is usually characterized through medical imaging studies, namely in ultrasound scoop. There is some variability associated with the performance of the ultrasound studies, which is very dependent on the equipment used, but also on the study protocol, on the equipment used, as well as on the experience and preferences of the observer, what makes it difficult to select the most appropriate strategies to characterize tibial nerve biomechanics using ultrasonography. Therefore, this chapter aims to i) characterize normal and pathological nerve biomechanics and how these can be used to inform non-invasive interventions directed at restoring normal nerve function using joint movement and ii) to critically analyze measurement procedures, image characterization and its reliability characteristics.

This will be achieved by summarizing and discussing the findings of existing literature characterizing normal biomechanics of the tibial nerve and comparing the normal biomechanics of this nerve against its biomechanics in the presence of pathology and by synthetizing existing evidence on ultrasound applied in the study of different pathologies that can affect peripheral nerves, namely in their performance, as well as the development of new procedures and technologies for a better nerve biomechanics characterization. We will also discuss the clinical implications of our findings, in particular for the use of neural mobilization, a technique commonly used by physiotherapists to treat pathology of the peripheral nerves.

Keywords: nerve biomechanics, ultrasonography, tibial nerve

NORMAL NERVE BIOMECHANICS

Nerve Strategies to Maintain Normal Function Despite Changes in Body Posture and Movement

Nerves are generally able to accompany body movements and postures and to accommodate the forces that these impose while maintaining a normal function. Forces acting on the nerves during body movements and posture could be tensile, shear or compressive. A variety of mechanisms make it possible for the peripheral nervous structures to adapt to the forces imposed. They glide in relation to adjacent structures, a mechanism that is named excursion; and the internal fascicules that constitute each nerve, slide against each other in deeper layers (intraneural gliding). Both internal sliding and gliding against adjacent structures make the normal gliding of the nerve possible [1]. They elongate increasing internal strain; and they have the ability to tolerate compression from adjacent structures [2]. Furthermore, the structural organization of nerves also facilitates normal function while allowing normal movement [2]. Examples of this are the considerable amount of connective tissue that surrounds the nerve and controls and facilitates nerve movement, while also protecting it; the fascicules that contain the nerve fibres follow an undulatory course with several branches that appear suited to accommodate movement and to promote dispersion of forces [3]; the myelin lamellae show the incisures of Schmidt–Lanterman whose function may be to provide metabolic support for the axonal Schwann cell but also to allow movement and stretching of the axon/myelin complex without damage [4]; the abundant blood supply provided by numerous arterial branches of different origins, which have a coiled structure to minimize the impact of movement on the normal blood supply, imperative for normal nerve function [5].

In addition to these strategies intrinsic to the nervous system, there are additional ones extrinsic to the nervous system, which are believed to exist to protect nerves from excessive forces during body movements and postures. For example, it is believed that increased muscle activity is a protective reflexive mechanism aiming to prevent further motion of the segment and, consequently, avoiding forces acting on the nerves from reaching levels that could potentially cause damage [6]. In support of this argument are the studies showing increased electromyographic activity during movements that elongate nerves both in the lower and upper limb. For example, a previous study demonstrated that there is muscle activation during the straight leg raise (a neurodynamic test used to assess the sciatic nerve and its branches) when performed with ankle dorsiflexion (a sensitizing manoeuvre to the sciatic and tibial nerve), in the soleus, semitendinosus, tibialis anterior and vastus medialis at the first onset of symptoms and that muscle activation presents earlier if the ankle is in ankle dorsiflexion compared to when the ankle is in plantarflexion [7]. It has also been reported that performing the upper limb neurodynamic test biased towards the median nerve with side flexion of the neck (a sensitizing manoeuvre of the median nerve and brachial plexus) influenced both range of motion and muscle activity to a greater extent than when the neck is in a neutral position, i.e., induced further limitation of elbow extension and increased activity of the trapezius muscle [8]. These data supports the assumption that muscles contract to prevent movement and protect nerves from potential damage. Furthermore mobilization of the nervous system in patients with lumbosciatic pain has been shown to reduce eletromiographic activity of muscles in the lower limb [9].

Nerve Patterns of Movement and Strain in Response to Joint Motion

Nerve movement in response to body movement is not straightforward as quantity and direction of movement (i.e., gliding in relation to adjacent structures) is influenced by a variety of factors such as range of joint movement, distance of the moving joint to the nerve, position of joints adjacent to the moving joint, number of joints moving and whether joint movement stretches or shortens the nerve [10]. The shortening or stretching of the nerve is important for the direction of the nerve movement, as it glides towards the moving joint when the movement stretches the nerve and away from the moving joint when it shortens the nerve [2, 10]. Furthermore, it seems that different sequencing of joint movements, i.e., adding the same movements from the same joints in a different order, changes the pattern of nerve movement and strain. This is likely due to the fact that nerves do not seem to respond to joint movement in a uniform way: first nerves tend to lose their slack, smoothing the undulatory configuration of the nerve fascicles and progressively increasing gliding against the nerve bed and then elongating and increasing stiffness and internal pressure. Studies have shown that although there is no difference at the end position for strain and quantity of nerve excursion when quantity of joint range of motion is consistent between sequences, there are differences in the pattern of nerve biomechanics (how strain increases and nerve movement occurs) at the progressive stages of different movement sequences [7, 11]. Movement and strain are higher in the nerve segment that is nearer the joint that is being moved. It has been shown that tibial nerve strain near the ankle joint increases earlier and is maintained longer in regions closer to the ankle when the ankle is moved first in the movement sequence of the straight leg raise as opposed to when it is moved after hip flexion [12]. Furthermore, it has also been shown that signs and symptoms differ when the same joint movements are added in different order for the median nerve, being more marked in the distal part of the limb when the order of movements was from distal to proximal [13]. These findings suggest that the sequencing of joint movements affect the pattern of nerve response, which could then have an impact on the signs and symptoms reported by the patient. This knowledge could be used to personalise neurodynamic tests (tests used to identify a potential compromise of peripheral neural structures) to a specific patient if proved to improve the tests' sensitivity. A biomechanical rationale for changing the order of the components of neurodynamic tests so that the first component of the test is that nearer to where the nerve is potentially damaged exists [11]: it allows the targeted nerve segment to support higher strain levels for a longer time period and the joint to reach full range (joints that are moved later are less likely to reach full range). Nevertheless, further research is needed on the impact on nerves of different joint movement sequencing and whether it translates into higher levels of diagnostic accuracy.

Tibial Nerve Biomechanics in Response to Joint Movement

Studies characterizing how the tibial nerve responds to movement in living humans are scarce and they tend to characterize the excursion of the nerve in relation to adjacent structures only. Two studies assessed the tibial nerve gliding at the popliteal fossa in response to ankle dorsiflexion either performed alone [14] or simultaneously to neck extension [15]. The tibial nerve glided distally (towards the moving joint) in both studies. Nerve gliding in response to ankle dorsiflexion alone was assessed in side lying with the hip at approximately 20º and 60º flexion and mean values decreased with increasing hip flexion. The tibial nerve mean gliding was 2.2 mm when the hip was at 20º flexion and was 0.7 mm when it was at 60º flexion [14]. Tibial nerve gliding in response to ankle dorsiflexion performed simultaneously to neck extension was assessed in a seated position and induced a mean gliding of 5.2 mm [15]. Taken together, the results of both studies confirm for the tibial nerve what was previously said regarding general nerve excursion: that the position of adjacent joints have an impact on the nerve excursion produced by a specific joint motion and that adding simultaneously a movement that elongates a nerve and a movement that shortens it produces more excursion on that nerve than using only movements that elongates the nerve. In addition to these two studies, Hum et al. [16] characterized tibial nerve movement at the popliteal fossa during forward bending in healthy subjects. The mean range of lumbar spine and hip flexion was 80.2º and 33.6º, respectively, and for this amount of movement they reported a mean proximal excursion (excursion towards the moving joints) of 12.2mm. Carroll et al. [17] measured tibial nerve excursion at the ankle when the foot moved from 10° plantarflexion to 20° dorsiflexion on a weight-bearing standing position and reported nerve excursion to be of 3.0 mm.

A study reporting on stiffness of the tibial nerve measured using shear-wave elastography immediately proximal to the tarsal tunnel during the straight leg raise in response to different combinations of joint movement found that increased nerve stretch significantly alters shear-wave velocity in a manner consistent with an increase in stiffness [18]. Measurements were taken in three different positions: 1) hip neutral, knee flexed to 90° and foot neutral; 2) hip neutral, knee maximally extended and ankle dorsiflexed to end of range; and 3) hip in maximum flexion (40-90°), while maintaining maximum knee extension and ankle dorsiflexion (full straight leg raise). In position 1, the mean tibial nerve shear-wave velocity was 3.3

± 0.1 m/s; position 2 caused a significant 60.0 ± 6.0% increase in tibial nerve shear-wave velocity (mean = 5.2 ± 0.2 m/s), and in position 3, there was a further increase (136.0 ± 9.0% from position 1) in tibial nerve shear-wave velocity (mean = 7.6 ± 0.3 m/s). Further studies are needed that characterize the biomechanical response of the tibial nerve to the movement of different body segments. This is of particular relevance as it seems to be affected in individuals with pathology.

Changes in the Tibial Nerve Biomechanics in the Presence of Pathology

Changes in normal nerve biomechanics have been shown for several pathologies and nerves such as carpal tunnel syndrome, cervicobrachialgia or epicondylitis, suggesting a compromise of the adaptive mechanisms of the nervous system in these conditions [19]. Regarding the tibial nerve, in particular, individuals with type two diabetes seem to have a reduction of nerve elasticity even before the onset of diabetic neuropathy, which deteriorates in proportion to the severity of the neuropathy and affects nerve conduction [20]. Furthermore, the mean cross-sectional area of the tibial nerve in diabetic patients was larger than that in controls (patients with diabetes: 6.1 ± 0.1 mm^2; controls: 4.8 ± 0.2 mm^2), and increased with increased severity of the neuropathy. Both reduced nerve elasticity and increased nerve diameter are likely to have consequences on nerve biomechanics. Furthermore, it has already been shown that the pattern of nerve excursion is different in older people with diabetes when compared with young and asymptomatic controls [14]. These authors assessed tibial nerve excursion (longitudinal, tranverse and antero-posterior) in two different positions: i) the hip in 20° flexion, full knee extension and a relaxed ankle position and ii) hip flexion to the point the participant reported the first onset of any sensory response to movement (approximately 62º); participants then performed active ankle motions from plantar flexion (≥30°) to dorsiflexion (≥0°). Authors [14] reported that there was increased longitudinal (distal) excursion of the tibial nerve when the hip was at 20º flexion compared to 60º flexion both in healthy and diabetic participants. The nerve also moved medially and superficially, but these movements were not affected by hip flexion. They also found that despite similarities in the pattern of nerve movement between healthy and diabetic participants there was a significant decrease in the quantity of longitudinal nerve excursion in the group of participants with diabetes (0.8 ± 0.5 mm) when compared to healthy controls (2.2 ± 0.5 mm) and of superficial excursion (participants with diabetes: 1.0 ± 0.6 mm; controls: 3.7 ± 1.5 mm). This significant decrease of nerve movement in the group of patients with diabetes may be due to increased quantity or stiffening of connective tissue within the nerve. In contrast to previous studies, one study reported that the longitudinal sciatic nerve excursion at the posterior thigh during a modified straight leg raise does not differ between asymptomatic individuals and patients with spinal referred leg pain [21]. This may suggest that changes in the nerve biomechanics might depend on the pathology.

Using Nerve Biomechanics to Inform the Clinical Use of Non-Invasive Techniques to Assess and Treat Pathology of the Peripheral Nervous System

Knowledge on nerve biomechanics is used to inform non-invasive clinical strategies of assessment of the peripheral nervous system. The most well-known are neurodynamic tests, which use a combination of joint movements that elongate the nerves to assess how they respond to movement. These joint movements are added in a specific sequence and stop when patient symptoms first appear. In order to make a distinction regarding whether symptoms arise from musculoskeletal structures or from nerves (structural differentiation) a sensitizing manouvre is added. This is a joint motion that elongates the nerve and that is distant from the region where the symptoms are believed to originate. A change in symptoms when adding this distal component is believed to indicate that symptoms have origin in a peripheral nervous structure as opposed to a musculoskeletal structure. The combinations of joint movements used to assess can also be used to treat (neural mobilization). It is believed that this technique facilitates the mobility of the nervous system [22]. Neural mobilization can be used in a way that joint movements elongate the nerve (tensioning technique) or in a way that aims to maximize nerve excursion in relation to adjacent structures (gliding technique) [22]. The first consists of performing joint movements that elongate the nerve till patient symptoms appear and then using the joint movement distal to the region where the nervous structure is believed to be impaired to mobilize away from symptoms. The second consists of using at least two joints performing movement simultaneously in a way that while one movement elongates the nervous structure, the other shortens it. For example, the tibial nerve is commonly assessed using the straight leg raise, a test combining ankle dorsiflexion, knee extension and hip flexion. If the tibial nerve was believed to be affected around the ankle joint, a tensioning technique would use hip flexion, from the amplitude where symptoms arose to extension, while a gliding technique would combine hip and ankle movements (or other combination of at least 2 joints) and while the ankle was performing dorsiflexion the hip would go into extension. The larger the amplitudes used, the higher the nerve excursion and strain. Nevertheless, it is believed that tensioning techniques increase nerve strain more than gliding techniques while gliding techniques increase nerve excursion more than tensioning techniques without the potentially large increases in nerve strain [23]. As such, gliding and tensioning techniques may be indicated at different stages of a rehabilitation program. The biomechanics of the nervous system can be used to individualise treatments according to patients' signs and symptoms and to progress treatment. For example, excursion and strain of the tibial nerve is larger around the moving joint and progressively decreases as the distance from the moving joint increases; therefore using joints distant to where the nerve is believed to be affected and progressing to the joint proximal to the problem could be a way to gradually expose the nerve to increases in strain and excursion, facilitating its desensitization while minimizing the likelihood of exacerbating patients symptoms, particularly in an acute situation. The position of adjacent joints, the number of joints or the amplitude of joint motion used are other ways of decreasing or increasing strain and excursion [10]. Although there is biomechanical evidence to support this personalization of neural mobilization as these factors affect quantity of nerve excursion as well as the pattern of nerve excursion and strain development [10, 11, 14], there is no evidence that it shows better results than a more standardized way of mobilizing the nervous system.

A first systematic review on the effectiveness of neural mobilization has concluded that no firm conclusion was possible due to the reduced number and poor quality of included studies [15]. Since then a number of studies have been conducted and systematic reviews have shown more positive conclusions. A recent systematic review focusing on chronic musculoskeletal conditions and considering the outcome measures of pain and disability found a total of 40 studies. Authors concluded that neural mobilization is effective in reducing pain and disability in certain neuromusculoskeletal conditions: nerve-related low back pain, nerve-related neck and arm pain, tarsal tunnel syndrome, and plantar heel pain. In contrast, they also reported evidence to be insufficient to support the use of neural mobilization for carpal tunnel syndrome, post–lumbar surgery, and cubital tunnel syndrome [24]. Another systematic review on the effects of lower body quadrant neural mobilization in healthy and low back pain populations also concluded that neural mobilization has positive effects on flexibility of healthy individuals and on pain and disability in patients with low back pain [25]. A critical review on the effectiveness of neural mobilization in patients with spinal radiculopathy [26] offers a discussion on the potential mechanisms of neural mobilization. Based on previous evidence they suggest that neural mobilization, a mechanical stimulus, may have an impact on patients' signs and symptoms by i) increasing intraneural fluid dispersion and, consequently, preventing or reducing intraneural edema; ii) by inducing an hypoalgesic effect on C-fiber mediated pain at the dorsal horn; iii) reducing the concentration of inflammatory mediators involved in nerve pain and iv) reducing intra-neural and extraneural adhesions. The proposed mechanisms are based on the work performed by several authors in cadavers [27], rats [28, 29] and living humans [19].

Whether different ways of mobilizing the neural system have a different impact on nervous system function, i.e., whether a procedure that increases strain within the nerve versus a procedure that facilitates excursion have different effects on nerve function, is unclear as the literature comparing both techniques is scarce. However, existing studies seem to suggest that depending on the treatment aim one procedure might be better than the other. For example, Beltran-Alacreu et al. [30] compared the hypoalgesisc effects of neural gliding against neural tensioning: neck flexion, knee extension and ankle dorsiflexion (tensioning) versus craniocervical flexion plus ankle plantar flexion (gliding). Pressure pain thresholds were measured in the craniocervical region, in the neck and at the tibialis anterior and results suggest that neural gliding may have a wider hypoalgesic effect when compared to neural tensioning [30]. In contrast, a study comparing neural mobilization (gliding and tensioning) as an adjunct to static stretching of hamstrings on knee range of motion concluded that bot techniques were effective in increasing hamstring flexibility [31].

Medical Imaging in the Study of Peripheral Nerves

In medical imaging, the modalities with the best results in the study of the peripheral nerves are Magnetic Resonance (MR) and Ultrasound (US). Concerning the radiography modality, it may contribute to the identification of indirect pathological signs such as, for example, entrapment syndrome due to fractures or bone callus [32–34].

Computed tomography (CT) is rarely used for the study of peripheral nerves, but it can allow the differentiation of lesions that result in an increase or decrease in density and nerve size [35], it can also be useful for the identification of pathology of the vertebral column, namely intra-extra-foraminal pathology [36] and it aids in the diagnosis of some entrapment syndromes caused by tumours, bone pathology or vascular disease, tumors of the peripheral nerves and neurofibromatosis, in addition to being able to provide an accurate staging of neurofibromas, and related bone deformities [36]. Despite the usefulness of CT in the study of tumors of the peripheral nervous system [37] as often the nerve trunks are wide and well-visualized, this imaging modality may be inadequate for the identification of pathological changes in the nerve micro-structure [38].

Table 1 represents the advantages and disadvantages of different medical imaging modalities in the study of peripheral nerves [39].

Table 1. Advantages and disadvantages of different medical imaging modalities (adapted from [39])

Imaging Modality	Advantages	Disadvantages
Computed Tomography (CT)	Good spatial resolution, excellent bone contrast, large field of view, volume acquisition with multiplanar reconstructions (MPR), readily available, quickly performed, interventional guiding for diagnostic and therapeutic procedures.	Irradiation, poor contrast resolution, occasionally requires iodinated contrast injection, generally provides only indirect information on PNS disease.
Magnetic Resonance (MR)	Excellent contrast resolution, very good spatial resolution, three-dimensional planes, no limitation in examining deep structures, good investigation of muscle mass (signs of denervation), research and development potential, investigation is less operator dependent.	Contraindications to MR, availability and appointments delays, high cost, static investigation, occasionally performed in un-physiological positions, limited field of view and long acquisition time.
Ultrasound (US)	Excellent spatial resolution, no contra indications, dynamic investigations possible, investigation of a large part of the nerve path, interventional ultrasound with diagnostic and therapeutic procedures, readily available and low cost.	Operator dependent, relatively long learning curve, poor contrast resolution, limitations in some deep or difficult to access anatomical areas.

Regarding the MR acuity for the diagnosis of peripheral nerve pathology, significant heterogeneity is identified. A hypersignal in MR studies using T2-weighted or STIR, along with increased nerve width and nerve flattening were the significant imaging findings identified in peripheral nerve MR studies [40]. The use of high-frequency transducers (10 to 17 MHz or more) makes it possible to view most of the trunks of peripheral nerves, such as the radial, median or tibial nerve [41]. MR and US imaging modalities show peripheral nerves and may reveal their size and internal structure; however, ultrasound presents the advantages of being able to perform a dynamic examination and evaluate segments of long nerves in a short time, non-invasiveness and being a low cost modality well accepted by patients [34].

US is a very important imaging modality for the study of peripheral nerves, and it can complement other imaging modalities, namely in studies of small-diameter nerves as cutaneous nerves or in the case of diffuse neuropathies the ultrasound allows the visualization of the trunk of long nerves and their branches [42].

The Ultrasonography in the Study of Peripheral Nerves: From Acquisition to Visualization

Although the visualization of the peripheral nerves using US still presents challenging difficulties that need to be overcome, the development of high-resolution sonography equipment has allowed the visualization and study of most peripheral nerves on a routine basis [43], namely the use of high-frequency linear transducers along with the use of appropriate depth and focal zones contributes to a significant increase in the quality of peripheral nerves US imaging [44]. In fact, the development of linear high-frequency transducers has confirmed their advantages when studying peripheral nerves [40, 45–48]. On the other hand, US is a well-tolerated medical imaging modality capable of producing images of peripheral nerves, as well as of performing dynamic and functional studies at relatively low cost [49].

The use of ultrasonography in patients who cannot be submitted to other types of imaging studies has been showing its importance for peripheral nerves characterization and analysis [48]. Technological development, in particular of high-frequency transducers (15 MHz or more), have contributed to increase the sensitivity of tools such as Doppler, and have lead to morphological and dynamic studies of the nerves, as well as to studies on its vascularization. For example, virtually all segments of the median, ulnar and radial nerves of the upper limb and many segments of the femoral, sciatic, peroneal (fibular) and tibial nerves of the lower extremity can be visualized using US [50].

The protocols for performing US studies are dependent on the purpose of the study and can be static or dynamic, and done while the patient is performing passive or active movement of the limbs. In recent years we have seen the proliferation of the use of ultrasonography in the study of peripheral nerves [42].

Depending on the type of transducer and focus area, the highest resolution is achieved at a depth of approximately 0.5-1.5 cm [51]. Peripheral nerves should be studied with high-frequency linear transducers. Currently, the most superficial nerves can be examined with the 17-5-MHz linear transducer. Deeper nerves should be studied with the 12-5-MHz transducer, and the most cursory nerves should be studied with higher frequencies (e.g., 18-8-MHz transducers). In some patients, the study of deeper nerves may be performed using 5-7 MHz curved transducer (e.g., when scanning the posterior thigh) [48, 52].

Nerves must be distinguished from other nearby structures to ensure correct identification. The muscles have a unique structure. Emerging in the echographic image as hypoechogenic structures and interspersed with small hyperechogenic layer corresponding to the connective fibrous tissue, they are easily distinguished from the nerves. The tendons sometimes arise adjacent to the nerves, moving proportionally to the movement of the joints and have higher anisotropy than the nerves.

Anisotropy refers to the reflection properties of tissue US. Tissues with low anisotropy tend to backscatter sound reflection, and those with high anisotropy tend to reflect the sound in such a way that the angle of incidence is equal to the angle of reflection, making them much brighter when the transducer is placed perpendicular to the nerve. On the other hand, the tendons are more homogeneously hyperechoic than the nerves. During the study execution, altering the echographic image acquisition angle, also changes the aspect of the tendon, varying between hyperechoic and hypoechogenic textures. When scanning longitudinally, reduced slippage of the nerves during flexion or active or passive extension of a limb is another way to differentiate them from tendons [53].

The Ultrasonography in the Study of Peripheral Nerves: From Visualization to Characterization

The studies of the peripheral nerves using US began to appear in the literature in the late 80's beginning of the 90's, especially with the works done by Fornage [54], Graif et al. [55], Sener et al. [56] and Silvestri et al. [57].

In US studies the peripheral nerve is analyzed in its axial plane where it appears as an oval structure, consisting of a network of hypoechogenic nervous fascicles separated by hyperechogenic septa comprised of collagen and connective tissue. In a longitudinal visualization, the peripheral nerves appear hypoechogenic, whereas the adjacent tendons appear more echogenic, compact and with a fibrillary texture [58].

Normal nerves are visualized with markedly echogenic tubular structures with parallel and hyperechogenic internal lines when in longitudinal acquisitions, and in honeycomb format in axial acquisitions. Peripheral nerves have a typical echo structure correlated with their histological structure which facilitates the differentiation between tendons and nerves [57].

The thickness of nerves can be quantified in longitudinal and cross-axial areas by evaluating the anteroposterior diameter and calculating the area of the nerve in an axial plane. Their size can be accurately measured in both longitudinal and transverse images and depends primarily on their function (e.g., motor, sensory, mixed) [59]. One of the factors to consider when assessing the peripheral nerve is its cross-sectional area (CSA) [60], which can be measured in axial images, whereas longitudinal excursion is measured in longitudinal images of the nerves. For correct measurement, the transducer must be held perpendicular to the nerve, with minimum pressure. The variability within a measure can be reduced using a mean of multiple measures. Measuring only within the echogenic edge of the nerve is the most commonly used approach [61]. However, it is important to note that the peripheral nerve caliber can be influenced by external factors such as temperature, body mass index, age, and gender of the patient [62].

Although many studies do not mention whether they include the hyperechogenic rim that circumvents the nerve, many investigators do not add it in their measurements since it is not always visible and is difficult to visualize [63]. However Nakamichi & Tachibana [64] have demonstrated that US measurements are reliable.

According to Kerasnoudis & Tsuvgoulis [65] the US examination of a peripheral nerve focuses mainly on the evaluation of its CSA, the variability of CSA along its anatomic course, echogenicity, vascularization and mobility. On the other hand, the echogenicity of the nerves is usually evaluated subjectively and is based on the experience of the operator. Some studies have introduced new techniques with the aim of helping the operator to quantify echogenicity in a reproducible way. Among pathological changes in the echogenicity of nerves, the most common are the reduction of fascicular echogenicity or selective hypertrophy of the nervous fascia [66, 67].

Regarding the differentiation between nerves, tendons and vascular structures, tendons have their beginning and end in muscular structures and vascular structures deform easily, namely by increasing the pressure of the transducer on them [43].

The change in dimension in the nerve is the most critical sign of the existence of pathology, so its characterization/measurement becomes essential [68]. The cross-sectional area and the swelling ratio can be evaluated in transverse/axial images, and the diameter can be measured in longitudinal acquisitions. Although the lesion site should be selected and evaluated by this procedure, it should be part of the CSA analysis with a minimum cross-sectional area at this location to guarantee an image acquisition perpendicular to the nerve.

When measuring nerve size, there may be some variability in the results. This variability may be associated with the inclusion of the echogenic rim in the nerve in the measurements. This variability can be reduced if several measurements are taken [61].

Alteration of Peripheral Nerve Mobility

One way of distinguishing tendons from nerves was mentioned by Fornage et al. [54] who found that nerves had a relative immobility during flexion and extension movements when compared with tendons and muscles. Silvestri et al. [57] also found that the hypoechogenic areas of the nerves were correlated with the fascicles and that the hyperechoic fundus was related to the epineurium. However, some studies underestimated the number of fascicles seen in microscopic analysis. According to these authors, this fact could be because these fascicles were only visualized when the probe was perpendicular to the nerve or due to little lateral resolution, which was evident when analyzing adjacent structures with similar echogenicity.

The knowledge of the regional and topographic anatomy is indispensable for the characterization of the tibial nerve. Identification of the tibial artery is important for the identification of this nerve. Once identified, the nerve could be viewed continuously in the proximal and distal directions. Although the nerve can be easily found and visualized according to the reference point, knowledge about the entire course is essential especially in patients who may present a variant of normal anatomy or with pathological changes, namely abnormal swelling ratio.

The swelling ratio is the relationship between the cross-sectional area of the nerve at the largest site and that of an unaffected site. This measure may improve the diagnostic accuracy for entrapment neuropathy in studies of patients with polyneuropathy with a diffuse increase in nerve size (e.g., patients with polyneuropathy or obesity) [69]. Another potentially useful parameter for assessing focal nerve compression is flattening ratio, which is defined as the ratio between the largest and smallest nerve diameter for example when the affected nerve presents a change in its shape [65].

To study the degree of vascularization of the peripheral nerves in neuropathy situations, a new form of vascularization quantification has been developed. It is possible to document the correlation, for example, between the severity of a carpal tunnel syndrome and the degree of hypervascularization [70]. However, the results of using this technique can be influenced by external factors such as temperature and sympathetic limb tone. Nerve vascularization, can be evaluated using color Doppler. In typical situations, the peripheral nerves do not present color Doppler signal. The presence of color represents the intraneural blood flow and is synonymous with the presence of pathtology (mainly as a result of an inflammatory process or compression) [65]. In this scoop, Ghasemi-Esfe and colleagues [70] developed an image processing method to quantify the degree of intraneural vascularization and found that the degree of intraneural vascularization measured has a high correlation with the condition severity corroborated with the electrodiagnostic test. Also Hough et al. [71] developed an application for evaluating longitudinal movement of peripheral nerves based on Doppler and concluded that spectral Doppler ultrasound may provide a useful method for noninvasive quantification of longitudinal nerve motion.

Kelle et al. [72], in the work performed aiming to evaluate the correlation between CSA of the peripheral nerves and the existence of peripheral diabetic neuropathy, concluded that ultrasound is a sensitive medical diagnostic modality to arrest the existence of peripheral diabetic neuropathy but does not indicate the severity of the disease.

The position of the structures and the amplitude of the articular mobilization may contribute to the alteration of the dimensions of the peripheral nerves. For example, Beekman et al. [73] recommended the study of the ulnar nerve in extension and elbow flexion at 90º since flexion greater than 90º promote a decrease in the size of the ulnar nerve in its axial/transverse plane. Also Kasehagen et al. [74] quantified the longitudinal displacement of the radial nerve during various active and passive movements of the wrist in healthy participants and concluded that real-time ultrasound is a reliable, cost-effective and in vivo method for analysis of the radial nerve excursion.

CONCLUSION

In conclusion, biomechanics of the peripheral nerves in general and of the tibial nerve in particular, are complex and need to be further characterized, especially for pathologic conditions. The ultrasound is a reliable, well accepted and relatively low cost imaging technique that could be used to shed further light both on peripheral nerve biomechanics and on its usefulness as a diagnostic indicator for some pathologies.

REFERENCES

[1] Rempel D, Dahlin L. Biological Response of Peripheral Nerves to Loading: Pathophysiology of Nerve Compression Syndromes and Vibration Induced Neuropathy. In: *Work-Related Musculoskeletal Disorders: Report, Workshop Summary, and Workshop Papers*. National Research Council (US) Steering Committee for the Workshop on Work-Related Musculoskeletal Injuries: The Research Base., eds. Washington: National Academies Press; 1999.

[2] Topp K, Boyd BS. Structure and Biomechanics of Peripheral Nerves: Nerve Responses to Physical Stresses and Implications for Physical Therapist Practice. *Phys Ther*. 2006;86:92-109.

[3] Gifford L. Neurodynamics. In: Pitt-Brooke, ed. *Rehabilitation of Movement: Theoretical bases of clinical practice*. London: Saunders; 1997:159-195.

[4] King R. Microscopic anatomy: normal structure. *Handb Clin Neurol*. 2013;115:7-27.

[5] Ugrenovic SZ, Jovanovic ID, Kovacevic P, Simic T. Similarities and Dissimilarities of the Blood Supplies of the Human Sciatic, Tibial and Common Peroneal Nerves. *Clinical Anatomy.* 2013;882:875-882.

[6] Gifford L. *The nerve root*. Cornwall: CNS Press; 2014.

[7] Boyd BS, Wanek DL, Gray AT, Topp PKS. Mechanosensitivity of the Lower Extremity Nervous System During Straight-Leg Raise Neurodynamic Testing in Healthy Individuals. *JOSPT*. 2009;39 (11):780-790.

[8] Heide B Van Der, Allison GT, Zusman M. Original article Pain and muscular responses to a neural tissue provocation test in the upper limb. *Man Ther.* 2001;6:154-162.

[9] Horment-Lara G, Cruz-Montecinos C, Núñez-Cortés R, Letelier-Horta P, Henriquez-Fuentes L. Onset and maximum values of electromyographic amplitude during prone hip extension after neurodynamic technique in patients with lumbosciatic pain: A pilot study. *J Bodyw Mov Ther*. 2016;20(2):31623.

[10] Silva A, Manso A, Andrade R, Domingues V, Piedade M, Silva AG. Clinical Biomechanics Quantitative in vivo longitudinal nerve excursion and strain in response to joint movement : A systematic literature review. *Clin Biomech. 2014;29(8):839-47.*

[11] Nee RJ, Yang C, Liang C, Tseng G, Coppieters MW. Impact of order of movement on nerve strain and longitudinal excursion : A biomechanical study with implications for neurodynamic test sequencing. *Man Ther*. 2010;15(4):376-381.

[12] Boyd BS, Topp KS, Coppieters MW. Impact of Movement Sequencing on Sciatic and Tibial Nerve Strain and Excursion During the Straight Leg Raise Test in Embalmed Cadavers. *J Orthop Sports Phys Ther.* 2013;43(6):398-403.

[13] Zorn P, Shacklock M, Trott P, Hall R. The effect of sequencing the movements of the upper limb tension test on the area of symptom production. In: Jull G, ed. *Manipulative Physiotherapist's Association of Australia 9th Biennial Conference*. Queensland; 1995:166e-167.

[14] Boyd BS, Gray AT, Dilley A, Wanek L, Topp KS. The pattern of tibial nerve excursion with active ankle dorsiflexion is different in older people with diabetes mellitus. *Clin Biomech*. 2012;27(9):967-71.

[15] Ellis R, Hing W. Neural mobilization: a systematic review of randomized controlled trials with an analysis of therapeutic efficacy. *J Man Manip Ther*. 2008;16(1):8-22.

[16] Hum GL, Ttenborough AS, Arsden JF, Ough AD. *Tibial nerve excursion during lumbar spine and hip flexion measured with diagnostic ultrasound*. 2013;39(5):784-790.

[17] Carroll M, Yau J, Rome K, Hing W. Measurement of tibial nerve excursion during ankle joint dorsiflexion in a weight-bearing position with ultrasound imaging Measurement of tibial nerve excursion during ankle joint dorsiflexion in a weight-bearing position with ultrasound imaging. *J Foot Ankle Res*. 2012;5(1):5.

[18] KaKantarci F, Ustabasioglu F, Delil S, et al. Median nerve stiffness measurement by shear wave elastography: a potential sonographic method in the diagnosis of carpal tunnel syndrome. *EUr Radiol*. 2014;24(2):434-40.

[19] Beneciuk J, Bishop M, George S. Effects of upper extremity neural mobilization on thermal pain sensitivity: a sham-controlled study in asymptomatic participants. *J Orthop Sport Phys Ther*. 2009; 39(6):428-38.

[20] Ishibashi F, Taniguchi M, Kojima R, Kawasaki A, Kosaka A, Uetake H. Elasticity of the tibial nerve assessed by sonoelastography was reduced before the development of neuropathy and further deterioration associated with the severity of neuropathy in patients with type 2 diabetes. *J Diabetes Investig*. 2016;7(3):404-12.

[21] Ridehalgh C, Moore A, Hough A. Sciatic nerve excursion during a modified passive straight leg raise test in asymptomatic participants and participants with spinally referred leg pain. *Man Ther*. 2015;20(4):5649.

[22] Butler D. *The sensitive nervous system*. Adelaide: Noigroup Publications; 2000.

[23] Coppieters M, Andersen L, Johansen R, et al. Excursion of the Sciatic Nerve During Nerve Mobilization Exercises: An In Vivo Cross-sectional Study Using Dynamic Ultrasound Imaging. *J Orthop Sport Phys Ther*. 2015;45(10):731-7.

[24] Basson A, Olivier B, Ellis R, Coppieters M, Stewart A, Mudzi W. The Effectiveness of Neural Mobilization for Neuromusculoskeletal Conditions: *A Systematic Review and Meta-analysis*. 2017;47(1401).

[25] Neto T, Freitas SR, Marques M, Gomes L, Andrade R. Musculoskeletal Science and Practice Effects of lower body quadrant neural mobilization in healthy and low back pain populations : A systematic review and meta-analysis. *Musculoskelet Sci Pract*. 2017;27:14-22.

[26] Efstathiou MA, Stefanakis M, Savva C, Giakas G. ScienceDirect Effectiveness of neural mobilization in patients with spinal radiculopathy : A critical review. *J Bodyw Mov Ther*. 2015; 19(2):205-212.

[27] Brown C, Gilbert K, Brismee J-. M, Sizer P, James C, Smith P. The effects of neurodynamic mobilization on fluid dispersion within the tibial nerve at the ankle: an unembalmed cadaveric study. *J Man Manip Ther*. 2011;19.

[28] Bertolini GRF, Silva TS, Trindade DL, Carvalho AR. Neural mobilization and static stretching in an experimental sciatica model – an experimental study. *Brazilian Journal of Physical Therapy*. 2009;13(6):2-7.

[29] Santos FM, Silva JT, Giardini AC, et al. Neural mobilization reverses behavioral and cellular changes that characterize neuropathic pain in rats. *Mol Pain*. 2012;8(1):57.

[30] Beltran-alacreu H, Jiménez-sanz L, Carnero JF, Touche R La. Comparison of Hypoalgesic Effects of Neural Stretching vs Neural Gliding: A Randomized Controlled Trial. *J Manipulative Physiol Ther*. 2015;38(9):644-652.

[31] Sharma S, Balthillaya G, Rao R, Mani R. Physical Therapy in Sport Short term effectiveness of neural sliders and neural tensioners as an adjunct to static stretching of hamstrings on knee extension angle in

healthy individuals : A randomized controlled trial. *Phys Ther Sport*. 2016;17:30-37.

[32] Samson P. Le syndrome du canal carpien. [Carpal tunnel syndrome] *Chir Main*. 2004;23(Supp. 1):S165-S177.

[33] Roulot E. Les syndromes canalaires autour du coude et de l'avant-bras. Partie 2: nerf radial et nerf médian. [Canal syndromes around the elbow and forearm. Part 2: Radial nerve and median nerve.] *Rev Rhum*. 2007;74(4):365-370.

[34] Bianchi S. Ultrasound of the peripheral nerves. *Jt Bone Spine*. 2008;75(6):643-649.

[35] Alexandre A, di Paola F, di Toma F, Cisotto P, Billeci D, Carteri A. Computed Tomography in Peripheral Nerve Pathology. In: *Peripheral Nerve Lesions*. Berlin, Heidelberg: Springer Berlin Heidelberg; 1990:201-203.

[36] Lecouvet F, Cosnard G. Conflit disco-radiculaire et diagnostic differentiel. [Disco-radicular conflict and differential diagnosis.] *J Radiol*. 2007;88(10):1337.

[37] Pilavaki M, Chourmouzi D, Kiziridou A, Skordalaki A, Zarampoukas T, Drevelengas A. Imaging of peripheral nerve sheath tumors with pathologic correlation. *Eur J Radiol*. 2017;52(3):229-239.

[38] Floch H, Naux E, Dang CP, Dupas B, Pinaud M. Computed Tomography Scanning of the Sciatic Nerve Posterior to the Femur: Practical Implications for the Lateral Midfemoral Block. *Reg Anesth Pain Med*. 2003;28(5).

[39] Kwee RM, Chhabra A, Wang KC, Marker DR, Carrino JA. Accuracy of MRI in Diagnosing Peripheral Nerve Disease: A Systematic Review of the Literature. *Am J Roentgenol*. 2014;203(6):1303-1309.

[40] Ellis JRC, McNally EG, Scott PM. Ultrasound of peripheral nerves. *Imaging*. 2002;14(3):217-222. doi:10.1259/img.14.3.140217.

[41] Ohana M, Moser T, Moussaou A, et al. Current and future imaging of the peripheral nervous system. *Diagn Interv Imaging*. 2014.

[42] Kowalska B, Sudoł-Szopińska I. Normal and sonographic anatomy of selected peripheral nerves. Part I: Sonohistology and general

principles of examination, following the example of the median nerve. *J Ultrason*. 2012;12(49):120-30.

[43] Gruber H, Kovacs P. *Sonographic Anatomy of the Peripheral Nervous System BT - High-Resolution Sonography of the Peripheral Nervous System.* In: Peer S, Bodner G, eds. Berlin, Heidelberg: Springer Berlin Heidelberg; 2008:15-41.

[44] Lawande AD, Warrier SS, Joshi MS. Role of ultrasound in evaluation of peripheral nerves. *Indian J Radiol Imaging*. 2014;24(3):254-258. doi:10.4103/0971-3026.137037.

[45] Stuart RM, Koh ESC, Breidahl WH. Sonography of Peripheral Nerve Pathology. *Am J Roentgenol*. 2004;182(1):123-129.

[46] Drapé JL, Guerini H, Feydy A, Chevrot A. Imagerie des syndromes canalaires du poignet. *J Radiol*. 2007;88(10):1368.

[47] Kotevoglu N, Gülbahce-Saglam S. L'échographie dans le diagnostic du syndrome du canal carpien : valeur intrinsèque et comparaison avec l'évaluation clinique. [Ultrasound in the diagnosis of carpal tunnel syndrome: intrinsic value and comparison with clinical evaluation.] *Rev Rhum*. 2005;72(3):221-225.

[48] Brown JM, Yablon CM, Morag Y, Brandon CJ, Jacobson JA. US of the Peripheral Nerves of the Upper Extremity: A Landmark Approach. *Radio Graphics*. 2016;36(2):452-463. doi:10.1148/rg.2016150088.

[49] Vlassakov K V, Sala-Blanch X. Chapter 16 - *Ultrasound of the Peripheral Nerves A2* - Tubbs, R. Shane. In: Rizk E, Shoja MM, Loukas M, Barbaro N, Spinner RJBT-N and NI, eds. San Diego: Academic Press; 2015:227-250.

[50] Suk JI, Walker FO, Cartwright MS. Ultrasound of Peripheral Nerves. *Curr Neurol Neurosci Rep*. 2013;13(2):328.

[51] Kopf H, Loizides A, Mostbeck G, Gruber H. Diagnostic Sonography of Peripheral Nerves: Indications, Examination Techniques and Pathological Findings. *Ultraschall Med*. 2011;32(3):242-63 2011.

[52] Hammer MR, Brandon CJ, Jacobson JA. US of the Peripheral Nerves of the Lower Extremity : A Landmark Approach. *RadioGraphics*. 2016;36:1-15.

[53] Suk JI, Walker FO, Cartwright MS. Ultrasonography of peripheral nerves. *Curr Neurol Neurosci Rep*. 2013.

[54] Fornage BD. Peripheral nerves of the extremities: imaging with US. *Radiology*. 1988;167(1):179-182.

[55] Graif M, Seton A, Nerubai J, Horoszowski H, Itzchak Y. Sciatic nerve: sonographic evaluation and anatomic-pathologic considerations. *Radiology*. 1991;181(2):405-408.

[56] Sener RN, Alper H, Ozturk L, Ozer H, Falakali S. Retroperitoneal part of the femoral nerve. *Neuroradiology*. 1991;33(2):159-161.

[57] Silvestri E, Martinoli C, Derchi LE, Bertolotto M, Chiaramondia M, Rosenberg I. Echotexture of peripheral nerves: correlation between US and histologic findings and criteria to differentiate tendons. *Radiology*. 1995;197(1):291-296.

[58] Martinoli C, Bianchi S, Derchi LE. Ultrasonography of peripheral nerves. *Semin Ultrasound, CT MRI*. 2000;21(3):205-213.

[59] Heinemeyer O, Reimers CD. Ultrasound of radial, ulnar, median, and sciatic nerves in healthy subjects and patients with hereditary motor and sensory neuropathies. *Ultrasound Med Biol*. 1999; 25(3):481-485.

[60] Duncan I, Sullivan P, Lomas F. Sonography in the diagnosis of carpal tunnel syndrome. *Am J Roentgenol*. 1999;173(3):681-684.

[61] Roll SC, Case-Smith J, Evans KD. Diagnostic Accuracy of Ultrasonography VS. Electromyography in Carpal Tunnel Syndrome: A Systematic Review of Literature. *Ultrasound Med Biol*. 2011;37(10):1539-1553.

[62] Cartwright MS, Passmore L V, Yoon J-S, Brown ME, Caress JB, Walker FO. Cross-sectional area reference values for nerve ultrasonography. *Muscle Nerve*. 2008;37(5):566-571.

[63] Nakamichi K-I, Tachibana S. Ultrasonographic measurement of median nerve cross-sectional area in idiopathic carpal tunnel syndrome: Diagnostic accuracy. *Muscle Nerve*. 2002;26(6):798-803.

[64] Nakamichi KI, Tachibana S. Enlarged median nerve in idiopathic carpal tunnel syndrome. *Muscle Nerve*. 2000;23(11):1713-8.

[65] Kerasnoudis A, Tsivgoulis G. Nerve Ultrasound in Peripheral Neuropathies: A Review. *J Neuroimaging*. 2015;25(4):528-38 2015.

[66] Boom J, Visser LH. Quantitative assessment of nerve echogenicity: Comparison of methods for evaluating nerve echogenicity in ulnar neuropathy at the elbow. *Clin Neurophysiol*. 2012;123(7):1446-1453.

[67] Tagliafico A, Tagliafico G, Martinoli C. Nerve Density: A New Parameter to Evaluate Peripheral Nerve Pathology on Ultrasound. Preliminary Study. *Ultrasound Med Biol*. 2010;36(10):1588-1593.

[68] Duncan I, Sullivan P, Lomas F. Sonography in the diagnosis of carpal tunnel syndrome. *Am J Roentgenol*. 1999;173(3):681-684.

[69] Shik Yoon J, Walker FO, Cartwright M. Ultrasonographic swelling ratio in the diagnosis ulnar neuropathy at elbow. *Muscle & Nerve*; 2008. 38(4):1231-1235.

[70] Ghasemi-Esfe AR, Khalilzadeh O, Vaziri-Bozorg SM, et al. Color and Power Doppler US for Diagnosing Carpal Tunnel Syndrome and Determining Its Severity: A Quantitative Image Processing Method. *Radiology*. 2011;261(2):499-506.

[71] Hough AD, Moore AP, Jones MP. Measuring longitudinal nerve motion using ultrasonography. *Man Ther*. 2000;5(3):173-180.

[72] Kelle B, Evran M, Balli T, Yavuz F. Diabetic peripheral neuropathy: Correlation between nerve cross-sectional area on ultrasound and clinical features. *J Back Musculoskelet Rehabil*. 2016;29(4):717-722.

[73] Beekman R, Visser LH, Verhagen WI. Ultrasonography in ulnar neuropathy at the elbow: A critical review. *Muscle Nerve*. 2011;43(5):627-635.

[74] Kasehagen B, Ellis R, Mawston G, Allen S, Hing W. Assessing the Reliability of Ultrasound Imaging to Examine Radial Nerve Excursion. *Ultrasound Med Biol*. 2016;42(7):1651-1659.

In: Horizons in Neuroscience Research ISBN: 978-1-53613-286-1
Editors: A. Costa and E. Villalba

Chapter 5

DISINHIBITION, RESPONSE-INHIBITION AND IMPULSE CONTROL DISORDER IN PARKINSON'S DISEASE

Sara Palermo[1,*] ***and Rosalba Morese***[1,2,*]
[1]Department of Psychology, University of Turin, Italy
[1,2]Faculty of Communication Sciences,
Università della Svizzera Italiana, Lugano, Switzerland

ABSTRACT

Impulse Control Disorders (ICDs) are behavioral disturbances in which a person fails to resist the drive to behave in ways that result in distress or impaired social and occupational functioning (Grant et al., 2006). The incidence of ICDs in Parkinson's disease (PD) is as high as 20%. Dopamine agonists can induce alterations in those frontostriatal networks that manage reward and mediate impulse monitoring and control. Indeed, tonic stimulation of dopamine receptors may damage inhibitory control mechanisms and reward processing, while promoting compulsive repetition of behavior (Ray & Strafella, 2010). ICDs have, in

* Corresponding Author Email: sara.palermo@unito.it.
* Corresponding Author Email: moresr@usi.ch.

fact, been associated with depressed mood, disinhibition, irritability, and appetite disturbance (Pantone et al., 2006).

Moreover, many PD patients have difficulties with mental processing speed, response-inhibition, and shifting between different conceptual sets, suggesting frontal-executive dysfunction.

The neurocognitive approach considers two measurable executive functions from which ICDs can be detected: 1) response-inhibition, which neural substrate is located in the inferior portion of the prefrontal cortex; 2) integration of reward/punishment contingencies in individual choices, which neural substrate is located in the orbital-prefrontal cortex.

Establishing such a relationship between disinhibition and executive functions could potentially be helpful for therapeutic research and for the efficient targeting of symptom relief in PD. For this reason, we present the preliminary results of an fMRI study with the aim of exploring response-inhibition performance and the neural correlates of inhibition that varied on self-reported trait impulsivity.

This chapter will discuss the role of functional neuroimaging for research on ICDs and disinhibition in PD. Significant neuropsychological and neuroanatomical data will be highlighted and attention will be drawn to the concept of "motor impulsivity" in terms of "disinhibition of prepotent responses.

Keywords: disinhibition, Parkinson's disease, ICD, response-inhibition, fMRI, insula, ACC, pre-SMA, TPJ

INTRODUCTION

It is important to understand the elderly who present with disinhibition of mood and behavior. "Disinhibition" can be considered an "umbrella" term: it is a lack of restraint manifested in disregard for social conventions, impulsivity, and poor risk assessment. Disinhibition affects motor, instinctual, emotional, cognitive, and perceptual aspects with signs and symptoms similar to the diagnostic criteria for mania (Grafman et al., 2002).

Disinhibition syndromes present with a spectrum of mood and behavioral changes that range from inappropriate behavior to full-blown mania. Disinhibition syndromes that present for the first time are far more likely to be due to an associated physical etiology than the primary mania due to bipolar disorder (Starkstein & Robinson, 1997). Secondary mania refers to presentations associated with neurological/systemic disease, in the absence of a history of mood disorder, to which the elderly are more prone (Starkstein & Robinson, 1997). Indeed, a careful consideration of possible causes - such as bipolar I disorder, pharmacological treatment, or cognitive disorders - is essential for appropriate management.

About 15% of people with Parkinson's disease (PD) experience disinhibition or an Impulse Control Disorder (ICD). In a study by Schiehser and colleagues (2013), both patients and caregivers reported significantly more problems with patient apathy, disinhibition, and executive dysfunction postdiagnosis as compared to before PD diagnosis. Patients and caregivers did not differ in their ratings of patient apathy and executive dysfunction, but differed in terms of levels of patient disinhibition, with patients reporting more symptoms than caregivers (Schiehser et al., 2013). The authors concluded that clinicians should be especially cautious when interpreting reports about levels of patient disinhibition postdiagnosis and any retrospective reports about prediagnosis behavior, as such reports may be discrepant between patients and caregivers (Schiehser et al., 2013).

Disinhibition is found among people with PD, especially for people who are male, 60+ years old, take medication Pramipexole Dihydrochloride and have bladder disorder (US Food and Drug Administration report). In November 2017, thirty-one people with Parkinson's disease and disinhibition were studied by the FDA (report constantly updated on www.ehealthme.com) (see Figure 1). Considering the demographic characteristics of those with PD and who experienced disinhibition, 17.86% were women, while 82.14% were men. At the onset of symptoms, 14.29% of patients were between 40-49 years of age, 28.57% between 50-59 years, and the remaining 57.14% over the age of 60. Top co-existing conditions for these people were considered to be: pain (6.45%), muscle spasms (6.45%), bladder disorder (6.45%), suicide attempt (3.23%), and high-blood pressure (3.23%). The most common drugs taken by these people were Pramipexole Dihydrochloride (25.81%), Fentanyl (19.35%), Diazepam (19.35%), Kemadrin (12.90%), and Mirapex

(9.68%). The main symptoms associated with disinhibition in these PD patients were delusion (29.03%), aggression (22.58%), stress and anxiety (16.13%), dyskinesia (16.13%), and pathological gambling (12.90%). In most cases, behavior improves after withdrawal of the dopaminergic agent.

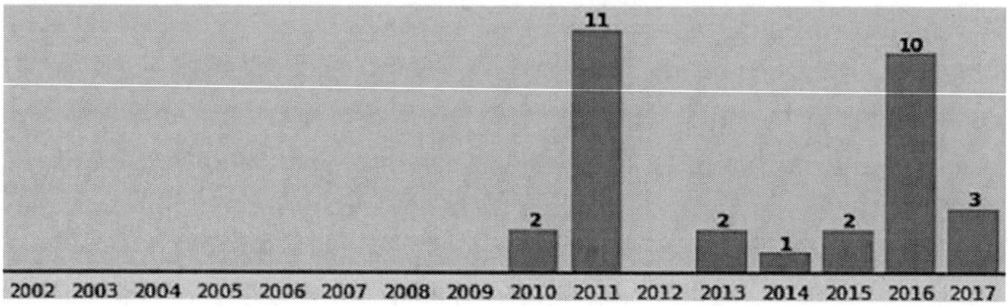

Figure 1. Trends in "disinhibition in Parkinson's disease" in FDA reports.

DISINHIBITION, IMPULSIVITY AND ASSOCIATED NEURAL SUBSTRATES

Disinhibition – the inability to inhibit inappropriate behavior - leads to social and emotional impairments, including impulsive behavior and disregard for social conventions.

As highlighted by Kocka & Gagnon (2014), *disinhibition is often considered a synonym for impulsivity.* As an example of this, in the manual "Neuropsychological assessment," Lezak and collaborators invite readers searching for disinhibition to see also impulsivity. Similarly, both impulsivity and disinhibition belong to the same domain of executive functions: initiation and planning (Constantinidou et al., 2012). Moreover, in a study evaluating conversational abilities in TBI patients, impulsivity and disinhibition constituted one factor representing impulsive or disinhibited conversational behaviors (Struchen et al., 2008).

For Luria (1969), however, disinhibition is the background on which euphoria, impulsiveness and inadequate emotional actions are superimposed.

Disinhibition syndromes may result from lesions to specific brain areas. Several studies in patients with closed head injuries, brain tumors, stroke lesions, and focal epilepsy have demonstrated a significant association between disinhibition and dysfunction of the right orbitofrontal and basotemporal cortices (Starkstein & Robinson, 1997). Based on their main connections with the dorsal regions related to spatial memory, somatosensation, and visuospatial functions, the orbitofrontal and basotemporal cortices may selectively inhibit or release motor, instinctive, affective, and intellectual behaviors elaborated in the dorsal cortex (Starkstein & Robinson, 1997). Thus, dysfunction of these heteromodal brain areas may result in dysfunction of this critical "decision-making" system and in disinhibited behaviors (Starkstein & Robinson, 1997).

A Neuropsychological Perspective on Impulsivity

Recent studies have extended beyond the idea of impulsivity being based in poorly planned actions, and have yielded to a broader definition that includes more cognitive functions (Antonelli, Ray & Strafella, 2011). In particular, according to Bechara's model (2000), two major processes linked to different neural networks and activated by different experimental paradigms have been defined: motor impulsivity and cognitive impulsivity. *Motor impulsivity* is described in terms of disinhibition of prepotent responses. *Cognitive impulsivity* is a more complex process, and is the result of a suppression of previously activated cognitive contents (Bechara, 2000; Antonelli, Ray & Strafella, 2011).

High levels of impulsivity are clinical features of several psychopathological and neurological disorders (Poletti, 2009). The neuropsychological approach offers useful tools to evaluate neurocognitive processes related to increased impulsivity (Poletti, 2009).

Two different components of impulsivity may be detected; one depends on response inhibition, an executive function based on the inferior portion of the prefrontal cortex and tested through tasks of the Go-NoGo type; the other depends on the integration of reward/punishment contingencies in individual choices, an executive function (EF) based on the orbital portion of the prefrontal cortex and tested through decision-making tasks.

EFs are instantiated in the dorsal, medial, and ventrolateral regions of the prefrontal cortex. However, the ventral region of the PFC, which includes the orbitofrontal cortex, plays more of an intermediary role between "hot" functions, like subjective valuation, and "cold" executive functions like response selection (Nelson, Jarchoa & Guyerb, 2016). Similarly, the anterior cingulate cortex (ACC) plays an important role in cognitive control, particularly in the context of affective experiences, learning, error monitoring, reward and awareness (Morese et al., 2016; Nelson, Jarchoa and Guyerb, 2016; Palermo et al., 2014; Palermo, 2017b). A number of studies have indicated that the ACC and vPFC play an important role in various aspects of social interaction (Morese et al., 2016). These regions might play a particularly important role in integrating social behavior with more traditional (cold) EFs (Nelson, Jarchoa & Guyerb, 2016).

Impulsivity has thus been associated with difficulty to inhibit behavioral responses and to alter choice behavior in response to fluctuations in reward contingencies (Poletti, 2009; Palermo et al., 2017c, 2017d).

FMRI Investigation of Disinhibition: Response-Inhibition and Impulsivity

Functional magnetic resonance imaging (fMRI) is a non-invasive technique for measuring and mapping brain activity. Its characteristic consists of high spatial and temporal resolution, important for recording dynamic changes in neural activity. It represents an indirect measurement based on the blood-oxygen-level dependent (BOLD) signal. During brain activation this technique detects the change from diamagnetic oxyhemoglobin to paramagnetic deoxyhemoglobin with the decrease in

MRI signal intensity. This means that when the increase in local metabolic demand in a specific brain area reflects an increased blood flow with decreased deoxyhemoglobin, the BOLD contrast increases (Niethammer et al., 2012).

fMRI is used in many studies to investigate the neural correlates involved in numerous motor, cognitive, disinhibition and impulsivity tasks and to gain a better understanding about how normal neural functions are altered in disease. Neuroimaging techniques can in fact be used to advance and increase our knowledge about structural and functional brain networks, and fMRI represents a powerful tool for investigating the functional neural correlates of diseases. In particular, in clinical RM applications this imaging instrument is used to expand our understanding of alterations related to motor, non-motor and cognitive symptoms (Ceballos-Baumann, 2003).

In neuroimaging studies there are two main types of design for conducting fMRI experiments: task and rest-related. The first measures the activations of regional cerebral functions triggered by different experimental task conditions associated with the BOLD signal, the second evaluates low-frequency spontaneous fluctuations in the BOLD signal when people are at rest without performing any specific task, in a baseline condition (resting-state fMRI, rs-FMRI).

With regard to the task design, two different types of experimental paradigms are used (Gore, 2003). The first is the so-called block design, in which stimuli (e.g., movements) and rest are presented alternately to the participants in blocks with a fixed long duration interval, for example 30 s for each one. In the second, which is usually referred to as an event-related design, the stimuli and baseline condition are alternated and randomized using a short duration interval, for example 3 s.

In clinical studies, the rs-fMRI technique is used to investigate functional connectivity associated with inhibition, motor and non-motor symptoms across patients' brain regions (Fox & Raichle 2007; Margulies et al. 2010, Prodoehl et al., 2014).

The event-related task design offers the advantage of recording the BOLD signal correlated to a single movement (Haslinger 2001) and avoiding the technical problems due to long acquisition times required with the block-design. The event-related fMRI design can be a powerful method to investigate movement disorders and disinhibition and impulsivity. A famous event-related task used for response inhibition paradigms is GO-NoGO, which involves the visual presentation of different stimuli with different frequencies in order to create conflicts in processing and in choosing between the response (GO) or no response (NoGO), i.e., response inhibition for NoGO trials. Braver and colleagues (2001) used this task condition to investigate the role of ACC activity during response inhibition, response selection, and target detection tasks. The authors instructed healthy participants to inhibit their response to infrequently presented NoGO stimuli (the letter 'X' = 17% frequency) and in the same context to respond to frequent GO stimuli (the 25 'non-X' letters = 83% frequency). Their results support the hypothesis that the ACC has a central role in detecting processing conflict when low-frequency responses are being executed. The data were analyzed using rapid event-related methods to evaluate the hemodynamic response time course for each stimulus. In this case of investigation of the low-frequency conditions, the high-frequency stimulus was considered as the baseline. Instead, in the equal-frequency conditions, one of the stimuli (GO or NoGO) can be defined as the arbitrary baseline. Several statistical models and software programs have been developed to process the large amount of neuroimaging data obtained by fMRI experiments, such as AFNI (Analysis of Functional Neuroimaging), SPM (Statistical Parametric mapping), BrainVoyager, FSL (FMRIB Software Library), REST (RESting-state fMRI data analysis Toolkit), etc. This aspect represents one of the biggest challenges in clinical MR applications.

From a clinical viewpoint, the use of fMRI in the study of inhibition and impulsivity may represent a potential help to better understand the clinical characteristics in the early diagnosis of patients.

DISINHIBITION AND IMPULSIVITY IN PARKINSON'S DISEASE

Parkinson's disease is the second most prevalent neurodegenerative disease in the world. It is characterized by resting tremor, bradykinesia, rigidity, postural instability. Secondary motor symptoms could be freezing of gait, micrographia, mask-like expression and unwanted accelerations. It can also be associated with autonomic dysfunctions, cognitive impairment, and neurobehavioral disorders, among which impulsivity and disinhibition disorders.

Disinhibition - the inability to inhibit inappropriate behavior - leads to social and emotional impairments, including impulsive behavior and disregard for social conventions.

In 2013, Fritsch and colleagues reported the first case showing that rapid, high-dosage increases in levodopa therapy can result in significant and detectable neuropsychological disinhibition. In particular, their PD patient exhibited an extreme increase in disinhibition when his levodopa dosage was rapidly increased, superimposed over a steady decline in processing speed that appeared related to progressive subcortical pathology (Fritsch et al., 2013). Moreover, "the psychologist also observed that the patient's thought processes seemed to be racing and he was unable to maintain focus in the face of distractors. He appeared disinhibited and impulsive, his reasoning was superficial, and his self-guided insight was poor. He was very apparently overwhelmed by stimuli in the room, unable to concentrate or maintain attention" (Fritsch et al., 2013, page 1).

In the same year, orbitofrontal (OFC) and right inferior frontal (IFC) cortex atrophy was shown to correlate with verbal disinhibition, while right nucleus accumbens atrophy was associated with response disinhibition (O'Callaghan et al., 2013). O'Callaghan et al. (2013) investigated the grey matter atrophy correlates of disinhibition in PD. Their results clearly show that grey matter atrophy in PD is related to inhibitory functioning across verbal and non-verbal measures of response disinhibition. Behavioral disinhibition effects were less severe in PD than in bvFTD, even though there were commonalities in the frontal and striatal areas that correlated with inhibitory dysfunction in both patient groups. In particular, PD patients' performance on inhibitory tasks correlated with grey matter atrophy - with verbal disinhibition corresponding to the frontal regions (medial OFC and right-sided lateral OFC/IFC) and response disinhibition corresponding to the right ventral striatal region (nucleus accumbens) (O'Callaghan et al., 2013).

These regions correspond to the fronto-striatal network purportedly affected by dopaminergic "overdose," which has also been implicated in impulsivity in PD via functional imaging and pharmacological manipulation studies (O'Callaghan et al., 2013). Indeed, the results obtained by O'Callaghan and colleagues (2013) suggest a structural component to impulsivity in PD, with atrophy in the OFC, right-IFC and right nucleus accumbens contributing to verbal and non-verbal response disinhibition. These findings support the suggestion by Milenkova and colleagues that factors other than dopaminergic therapy may mediate impulsivity in PD (Milenkova et al., 2011). Structural abnormalities in the OFC, right IFC and right nucleus accumbens are associated with failures in inhibitory control in PD, and thus may contribute to impulsive behaviors (O'Callaghan et al., 2013). Differences in grey matter atrophy may explain why some individuals are more vulnerable to the effects of treatment and go on to develop ICDs (O'Callaghan et al., 2013). Clinically, this would indicate that clinicians might need to take such atrophy into account, particularly OFC, when assessing risk factors for the development of impulsivity in PD (O'Callaghan et al., 2013; Palermo et al., 2017c, 2017d).

Clinical Features Associated with Disinhibition and Impulse Control Disorders in PD

ICDs are a heterogeneous class of disorders that are characterized by repeated and excessive performance of typically or initially hedonic behaviors (Pontone et al., 2006). There is an increasing awareness that ICDs can occur as a complication of PD and are associated with depressed mood, disinhibition, irritability, and appetite disturbance (Pontone et al., 2006). These behaviors can be socially devastating, but may be undiagnosed.

ICDs include behaviors such as pathological gambling, compulsive shopping, hypersexuality and compulsive eating. Other ICD-related behaviors seen less frequently include punding (stereotyped, repetitive, non-goal directed behaviors or excessive hobbyism) and dopamine dysregulation syndrome (compulsive PD medication overuse), and more recently hoarding, impulsive smoking, and kleptomania have been reported. It is not uncommon for individuals to have more than one ICD concurrently. Discrete symptoms of depressed mood, irritability, and appetite changes, in addition to disinhibition, are more likely to be present in PD-ICD than in PD alone (Pontone et al., 2006).

The reported occurrence of the primary ICDs associated with PD is extremely broad, with prevalence estimates ranging from 3.5% to 42.8% (Antonini et al., 2017). Several risk factors are considered: younger age at onset, male sex, single status, a family/personal history of addictive behaviors, dopamine agonist medication in combination with levodopa treatment, high doses of dopaminergic medication, longer disease duration, long duration of pharmacological treatments, and a personality profile characterized by impulsiveness (Bugalho & Oliveira-Maia, 2013; Antonini et al., 2017).

Dopamine and Neural Substrate of Impulse Control Disorders in PD

An association between ICDs and the use of dopamine agonists has been reported in the literature (Weintraub, 2008). Data suggest that risk factors for an ICD may include male sex, younger age or younger age at PD onset, a pre-PD history of ICD symptoms, personal or family history of substance abuse or bipolar disorder, and a personality style characterized by impulsiveness (Weintraub, 2008).

As reported by Weintraub (2008), "dopamine function, particularly within the mesocorticolimbic pathways, is critical in the mediation of reward and reinforcement behaviors. The brain regions most implicated in ICDs include the ventromedial and orbitofrontal regions of the prefrontal ortex, the ventral striatum (particularly the nucleus accumbens), and the amygdala, all of which are thought to mediate aspects of motivated behaviors underlying engagement in risky, compulsive behaviors. Finally, data suggest that alterations in cortico-striato-thalamo-cortical circuitry contribute to ICD behaviors, with projections coursing through the more ventral component of the striatum (including the nucleus accumbens) more implicated in urges and impulsive aspects, and those involving the dorsal striatum more implicated in motoric habits and compulsive aspects" (page S96).

Trait Impulsivity and Response-Inhibition in Parkinson's Disease. Preliminary FMRI Findings

Functional changes in the basal ganglia circuitry are responsible for the major clinical features of PD (Palermo et al., 2017c). The subthalamic nucleus (STN) has been regarded as a significant modulator of basal ganglia output and it has been studied because of its dual role in movement and in non-motor behaviors. In particular, the STN has been implicated in impulse control and the related construct of valence processing (Rossi, Gunduz, & Okun, 2015). Dopamine replacement treatment and dopamine-agonists have been implicated in impulse-control disorder development, since they can induce alterations in those fronto-striatal networks that manage reward and mediate impulse monitoring and control (Ray and Strafella, 2010).

Our case report (Palermo et al., 2017c) refers to a 51-year-old man (RL) with a 12-year history of Parkinson's disease, presenting motor fluctuations, and stable on 375 mg/day of levodopa. The subject was admitted to hospital for ascertainment as a candidate for deep brain stimulation surgery (MDS-UPDRS-III OFF=56; Hoehn-Yahr=2).

In 2014, the patient developed ICD symptomatology, including compulsive intake of sugary and high-fat foods, and video-game dependence. Grazing behavior and hyper-focus on in-game achievements interfered with the patient's everyday life. The neuropsychological assessment was performed in the best-on phase, immediately after the neurological examination and approval by the treating neurologist. The evaluation was based on the guidelines of the Task Force commissioned by the Movement Disorder Society to identify Mild Cognitive Impairment (Amanzio et al., 2014; Palermo et al., 2017a; 2017c). Neuroimaging data acquisition was performed on a 3T Philips Ingenia scanner. Images of the whole brain were acquired using a T1-weighted sequence (TR=4.8ms, TI=1650ms, TE=331ms, voxel-size=1×1×1mm3). Functional data were acquired using T2*-weighted EPI (TR=2.20s, TE=35ms, slice-matrix=64×64, slice gap=0.28 mm, FOV=24cm, flip angle=90°, slices aligned on the AC-PC line). During neuroimaging data acquisition, RL was asked to perform a response-inhibition ACC-sensitive task in which the subject had to respond to GO stimuli inhibiting the response to infrequent NoGO stimuli (Braver et al., 2001; Amanzio et al., 2013; Palermo et al., 2015). The paradigm we used is a prototypical task to measure the ability to inhibit an overpowering response. It involves two different sub-tasks: one requires a fast GO response, which has to be inhibited on a subset of trials that require a stop (or NoGO) response (Braver et al., 2001). RL had to respond to go stimuli (the letters "not-X" with a frequency of 83%) inhibiting the response to infrequent no-go stimuli (the letter "X" with a frequency of 17%). Every stimulus was shown for 250 ms with a 1 sec inter-stimulus interval. After scanning, the patient was asked to provide an estimate of the number of errors made in the experimental session. Image preprocessing was performed using SPM8. All functional images were spatially realigned to the first volume and anatomical images were co-registered to the mean image. The functional images were normalized to the MNI space and smoothed with an 8mm Gaussian Kernel. After preprocessing, we applied a General Linear Model to convolve the GO and

NoGO stimuli with canonical hemodynamic response function. The GLM consisted of a set of eight regressors: two categorical regressors, GO and NoGO, for inhibition ACC sensitive paradigm and six parametric regressors for motion extent. At the second level, to investigate the neural correlates of response-inhibition, we performed a one-sample t-test of contrast: NoGO vs. GO across all the participants using small volume correction [SVC] with a sphere of 10mm radius centered on the ACC according to the coordinates reported in Braver et al. (2001). This volume of interest encompasses the midcingulate zone, which has been shown to be specifically activated during tasks that require response selection and willful generation of motor behavior (Amanzio et al., 2013; Palermo et al., 2015). This sub-region of the ACC is located posterior to the genu of the ACC, anterior to the vertical plane passing through the anterior commissure (Amanzio et al., 2013; Palermo et al., 2015). In addition, to investigate which of the regions were associated with trait impulsivity, the degree of self-reported impulsivity was investigated in-group by regressing individual scores on the Barratt Impulsiveness Scale onto whole brain analysis, (FWE-corrected cluster $p<.001$).

The examination findings included the following: bilateral bradykinesia and tremor of the upper limbs. The remaining neurological examination was negative. The neuropsychiatric assessment revealed significant levels of anxiety. Although the patient exhibited a normal global cognitive profile, reaching normative scores on the screening tests, abnormalities were detected for performance on conceptualizing and response-inhibition tasks included in the Frontal Assessment Battery (Dubois et al., 2000).

The MRI showed no alterations in the brain parenchyma signal. However, the RL showed no response-inhibition abilities as measured by the GO-NoGO task and action-monitoring deficits (implying impaired error awareness). Moreover, fMRI acquisition revealed the absence of task-sensitive recruitment of the anterior cingulate cortex, medial prefrontal and orbitofrontal cortices for the NoGO versus GO contrast, signifying that a hypo-function of this network could be associated with ICD. A fronto-striatal and cingulo-frontal dysfunction may reflect

impairment of metacognitive-executive abilities (such as response-inhibition, action monitoring and error awareness) and promote compulsive repetition of behavior. Interestingly, impaired response-inhibition is an example of the motor/behavioral aspect of impulse control (Palermo et al., 2017c). A first contribution to the understanding of this data was provided by Li and colleagues (2008) who previously identified the rostral cingulate as the area underlying poor performance in a response-inhibition task in cocaine-addicted subjects, with greater impulsivity correlating with ACC hypo-functionality.

Having considered the important diagnostic/prognostic implications arising from this early work, a new cross-sectional study has been designed (Palermo et al., 2017d). To date, ten cognitively non-impaired patients with idiopathic PD receiving levodopa treatment, and presenting motor fluctuations have been enrolled. Consecutive outpatients were recruited at the Neurology Division of the Department of Neuroscience in Turin (Italy). They underwent a neurological evaluation, a neuropsychological assessment and were administered questionnaires on behavioral mood changes. The Barratt Impulsiveness Scale (BIS-11: Patton et al., 1995) provided an integrated measure of trait impulsivity. The BIS-11 is a questionnaire designed to assess the personality/behavioral construct of impulsiveness (Patton et al., 1995). It includes 30 items and three second-order factors (attentional, motor, and non-planning impulsiveness). During an fMRI acquisition, each subject performed the previously adopted GO-NoGO task (Braver et al., 2001; Amanzio et al., 2013; Palermo et al., 2015). Associations between the BOLD response of the whole brain during the response-inhibition task and trait impulsivity were investigated.

Our PD patients performed a response-inhibition task requiring the ability to inhibit overpowering responses while at the same time giving a continuous response to the GO stimulus. Intentional inhibition is considered as a cognitive control sub-component, which is a higher-order supervisory process, aimed at optimizing and modulating lower-order functions (Miller & Cohen, 2001). A significant association between higher impulsivity scores and worse performance was present ($p= 0.038$).

In this study, inhibitions of impulses to act were considered at the nexus between the decision to inhibit an action and the actual act of inhibition (Skaggs, 1929), which can be measured when an overpowering motor action is not performed or takes more time than usual. Not only does response-inhibition involve motor-related brain areas more widely than purely cognitive-inhibition, but it is voluntary and involves some degree of consciousness most of the time. Impulsivity may be secondary to executive function impairment: the co-occurrence of dysfunctional inhibitory processes and strong impulses, triggered and modulated by dispositional and situational variables, can lead to impulsive behavior (Hofmann et al., 2009). In line with the above consideration, we found a significant association between higher impulsivity scores and worse response-inhibition as measured by the NoGO/GO contrast (Palermo et al., 2017d).

The key aspect of our research is the direct investigation of the relationship between trait impulsivity measures and BOLD response. PD patients with higher scores on BIS-11 had greater activation of the bilateral presupplementary motor area (pre-SMA), bilateral anterior insula, right anterior cingulate cortex, and right temporal parietal junction (TPJ) during response-inhibition (see Table 1 and Figure 2). A massive recruitment of pre-SMA [*appropriate behavior selection*], ACC-AIC [*on-going event processing*], and TPJ [*attentional control*] would enable PD subjects with greater trait impulsivity to perform a Go/NoGO task with better results for the response selection (GO/NoGO) than for the response-inhibition per se (NoGO/GO). Taken together, these clinical findings suggest that execution of inappropriate motor responses reflects poor impulse control (Duque and Ivry, 2009). Impaired response-inhibition is an example of the motor/behavioral aspect of impulse control (Nemoda et al., 2011).

Our results suggest that a deficit in inhibitory processes ("disinhibition") may affect everyday life, causing impulsive conduct, which is generally detrimental for PD patients. The strong association between BIS-11 scores, MPFC, pre-SMA and TPJ suggests that greater engagement of that network was needed to maintain behavioral inhibition in more impulsive PD patients. Indeed, neuroimaging of brain activity during GO-NoGO tasks may be useful in characterizing the clinical profile while evaluating the treatment options. Indeed, response-inhibition assessment is thought to be particularly useful in order to better identify individuals at risk of developing ICD with dopaminergic medication.

Table 1. Regression analyses with questionnaire measures (FWE-corrected cluster p<.001)

BIS-11	MNI coordinates			Z-scores
	x	*y*	*z*	
Supplementary Motor Area	5	16	50	4.33
Supplementary Motor Area	-2	53	24	4.31
Anterior Insula Cortex	36	29	-2	3.99
Anterior Insula Cortex	-39	16	2	4.62
Anterior Cingulate Cortex	7	26	34	3.55
Temporal Parietal Junction	48	-39	30	4.42

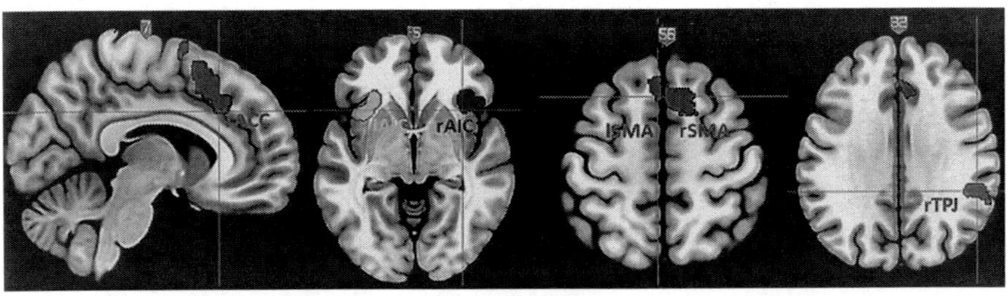

Figure 2. fMRI results for the regression analyses with BIS-11 measures (FWE-corrected cluster p<.001).

Conclusion

ICD has been associated with depressed mood, disinhibition, irritability, and appetite disturbance (Pontone et al., 2006). Moreover, many PD patients have difficulties with mental processing speed, response-inhibition, and shifting between different conceptual sets, suggesting frontal-executive dysfunction. The authors' hypothesis pointed out how behavioral addiction (i.e., motor impulsivity) is related with disinhibition of prepotent responses. Indeed, executive dysfunction in terms of response-inhibition could be a predisposing factor able to define the progression of ICD (Palermo et al., 2017c).

In our experience, fMRI response-inhibition tasks are useful for better characterizing the clinical profile while evaluating treatment options. A frontostriatal–cingulofrontal dysfunction may reflect impairment in metacognitive-executive abilities (such as response-inhibition, action monitoring and error awareness). Interestingly, impaired response-inhibition is an example of the motor/behavioral aspect of impulse control. Its assessment is believed to be particularly useful in the PD post-diagnostic phase, to better identify individuals at risk of developing ICDs with dopaminergic medication. Indeed, establishing a relationship between disinhibition and executive functions could potentially be helpful for therapeutic research and for the efficient targeting of symptom relief in PD. Theoretical models will be more effective if they integrate fMRI and neuropsychological data according to a neurocognitive approach to Parkinson's disease and ICDs.

References

Amanzio, M., Palermo, S., Zibetti, M., Leotta, D., Rosato, R., Geminiani, G., et al. (2014). Self-unawareness of levodopa induced dyskinesias in patients with Parkinson's disease. *Brain and cognition,* 90, 135-141.

Amanzio, M., Torta, D. M. E., Sacco, K., Cauda, F., D'Agata, F., Duca, S., et al. (2011). Unawareness of deficits in Alzheimer's disease: role of the cingulate cortex. *Brain: A Journal of Neurology,* 134(Pt 4), 1061-1076.

Antonelli, F., Ray, N., Strafella, A. P. (2011). Impulsivity and Parkinson's disease: more than just disinhibition. *J Neurol Sci.,* 310(1-2), 202-207.

Antonini, A., Barone, P., Bonuccelli, U., et al. (2017). ICARUS study: prevalence and clinical features of impulse control disorders in Parkinson's disease. *J Neurol Neurosurg Psychiatry,* 88, 317-324.

Bechara, A., Damasio, H., Damasio, A. R. (2000). Emotion, decision making and the orbitofrontal cortex. *Cereb Cortex,* 3, 295-307.

Braver, T. S., Barch, D. M., Gray, J. R., Molfese, D. L., & Snyder, A. (2001). Anterior cingulate cortex and response conflict: effects of frequency, inhibition and errors. *Cereb Cortex,* 11(9), 825-836.

Bugalho, P., Oliveira-Maia, A. J. (2013). Impulse control disorders in Parkinson disease: crossroads between neurology, psychiatry and neuroscience. *Behav Neurol.*, 547-557.

Ceballos-Baumann, A. O. (2003). Functional imaging in Parkinson's disease: activation studies with PET, fMRI and SPECT. *J Neurol.,* 250 (1), 15-23.

Constantinidou, F., Wertheimer, J. C., Tsanadis, J., Evans, C., Paul, D. R. (2012). Assessment of executive functioning in brain injury: Collaboration between speech-language pathology and neuropsychology for an integrative neuropsychological perspective. *Brain Inj.,* 26, 1549-1563.

Dubois, B., Litvan, I. (2000). The FAB: A frontal assessment battery at bedside. *Neurology,* 55(11), 1621-1626.

Duque, J., Ivry, R. B. (2009). Role of corticospinal suppression during motor preparation. *Cereb Cortex,* 19(9), 2013-24.

Fox, M. D., Raichle, M. E. (2007). Spontaneous fluctuations in brain activity observed with functional magnetic resonance imaging. *Nat Rev Neurosci,* 8, 700–711.

Fritsch, T., Hyde, T., Wallendal, M. S., Nausieda, P. A. (2013). L-DOPA-Induced Disinhibition in Parkinson Disease: More than Agonistic Behavior. *Biol Syst* 2: 115.

Grafman, J., Boller, F., Berndt, R. S., Robertson I. H., Rizzolatti, G. (2002). *Handbook of Neuropsychology*. Elsevier Health Sciences. p. 103. ISBN 978-0-444-50365-7.

Hofmann, W., Friese, M., Strack, F. (2009). Impulse and self-control from a dual-systems perspective. *Perpectives on Psychological Science,* 4, 162-176.

Kocka, A., Gagnon, J. (2014). Definition of Impulsivity and Related Terms Following Traumatic Brain Injury: A Review of the Different

Concepts and Measures Used to Assess Impulsivity, Disinhibition and other Related Concepts. *Behav Sci* (Basel), 4(4), 352–370.

Lezak, M. D., Howieson, D. B., Bigler, E. D., Tranel D. *Neuropsychological Assessment*. 5th ed. Oxford University Press; New York, NY, USA: 2012.

Li, C. R., Huang, C., Yan, P., Bhagwagar, Z., Milivojevic, V., Sinha, R. (2008). Neural correlates of impulse control during stop signal inhibition in cocaine dependent men. *Neuropsychopharmacology,* 33, 1798-1806.

Luria, A. R. Frontal lobe syndromes. In: Vinken P. J., Bruyns G. W. B., editors. *Handbook of Clinical Neurology*. North-Holland Publishing Company; Amsterdam, North Holland, The Netherlands: 1969. Volume 2.

Margulies, D. S., Bottger, J., Long, X., LV, Y., Kelly, C., Schafer, A., Goldhahn, D., Abbushi, A., Milham, M. P., Lohmann, G., et al. (2010). Resting developments: A review of fMRI post-processing methodologies for spontaneous brain activity. *Magma,* 23, 289–307.

Milenkova, M., Mohammadi, B., Kollewe, K., Schrader, C., Fellbrich, A., Wittfoth, M. (2011). Intertemporal choice in Parkinson's disease. *Movement Disorders,* 26(11), 2004-2010.

Miller, E. K., Cohen, J. D. (2001). An integrative theory of prefrontal cortex function. *Annual Review of Neuroscience,* 24, 167-202.

Morese, R., Rabellino, D., Sambataro, F., Perussia, F., Valentini, M. C., Bara, B. G., Bosco, F. M. (2016). Group Membership Modulates the Neural Circuitry Underlying Third Party Punishment. *PLoS ONE*, 11, 1-14.

Nelson, E. E. Jarchoa J. M., Guyerb, A. E. (2016). Social re-orientation and brain development: An expanded and updated view. *Developmental Cognitive Neuroscience,* 17, 118-127.

Nemoda, Z., Szekely, A., Sasvari-Szekely, M. (2011). Psychopathological aspects of dopaminergic gene polymorphisms in adolescence and young adulthood. *Neurosci Biobehav Rev.,* 35(8), 1665-86.

Niethammer, M., Feigin, A., Eidelberg, D. (2012). Functional Neuroimaging in Parkinson's Disease. *Cold Spring Harb Perspect Med,* 2(5), a009274.

O'Callaghan, C., Naismith, S. L., Hodges, J. R., Lewis, S. J., Hornberger, M. (2013). Fronto-striatal atrophy correlates of inhibitory dysfunction in Parkinson's disease versus behavioural variant frontotemporal dementia. *Cortex,* 49(7), 1833-43.

Palermo, S., Morese, R., Stanziano, M., Zibetti, M., Romagnolo, R., Sirgiovanni, S., De Faveri, L., Valentini, M. C., Lopiano, L. (2017d). Trait impulsivity and response-inhibition in Parkinson Disease. *An fMRI study*. BioRxiv doi: https://doi.org/10.1101/204768.

Palermo, S., Morese, R., Zibetti, M., Dematteis, F., Sirgiovanni, S., Stanziano, M., Valentini, M. C., Lopiano, L (2017c). Impulse control disorder and response-inhibition alterations in Parkinson's disease. A rare case of totally absent functionality of the medial-prefrontal cortex and review of literature. *Journal of Advanced Research*, 8(6), 713-716.

Palermo S. (2017b) Reduced self-awareness across pathologies: Involvement of the Anterior Cingulate Cortex. Eds Nova Science Publishers, Hauppauge, NY. In: AA.VV. *Horizons in Neuroscience Research* (Vol. 28). In A. Costa & E. Villalba (Eds.), Hauppauge, New York: Nova Science Publishers.

Palermo, S., Lopiano, L., Zibetti, m., Rosato, R. P., leotta, D., Amanzio, M. (2017a). A novel framework for understanding reduced awareness of dyskinesias in Parkinson's Disease. *Parkinsonism & Related Disorders* 39, 58-63.

Palermo, S., Cauda, F., Costa, T., Duca, S., Gallino, G., Geminiani, G., et al. (2015). Unawareness of bipolar disorder: the role of the cingulate cortex. *Neurocase,* 21(4), 438-447.

Palermo, S., Leotta, D., Bongioanni, M. R., & Amanzio, M. (2014). Unawareness of deficits in ischemic injury: role of the cingulate cortex. *Neurocase,* 20(5), 540-555.

Patton, J. H., Stanford, M. S., Barratt, E. S. (1995). Factor structure of the Barratt Impulsiveness Scale. *Journal of Clinical Psychology*, 51(6), 768-74.

Poletti, M. (2009). A neuropsychological perspective on impulsivity in Axis I disorders. *Giorn Ital Psicopat,* 15, 193-204.

Pontone, G., Williams, J. R., Bassett, S. S., Marsh, L. (2006). Clinical features associated with impulse control disorders in Parkinson disease. *Neurology*, 67(7), 1258-61.

Prodoehl, J., Burciu, R. G., Vaillancourt, D. E. (2014). Resting state functional magnetic resonance imaging in Parkinson's disease. *Curr Neurol Neurosci Rep,* 14(6), 448.

Ray, N., Strafella, A. P. (2010). Dopamine, reward, and frontostriatal circuitry in impulse control disorders in Parkinson's disease: insights from functional imaging. *Clin EEG Neurosci,* 41, 87-93.

Rossi, P. J., Gunduz, A., Okun M. S. (2015). The subthalamic nucleus, limbic function, and impulse control. *Neuropsychol Rev*, 25, 398-410.

Schiehser, D. M., Liu, L., Lessig, S. L., Song, D. D., Obtera, K. M., Burke Iii, M. M., Earl, S. R., Vincent F. J. (2013). Predictors of discrepancies in Parkinson's disease patient and caregiver ratings of apathy, disinhibition, and executive dysfunction before and after diagnosis. *J Int Neuropsychol Soc.,* 19(3), 295-304.

Skaggs, E. B. (1929). The major descriptive categories of inhibition in psychology. *Journal of Abnormal and Social Psychology*, 24, 310-317.

Starkstein, S., Robinson, R. (1997). Mechanism of disinhibition after brain lesions. *J Nerv ment Dis*, 185, 108-114.

Struchen, M. A., Pappadis, M. R., Mazzei, D. K., Clark, A. N., Davis, L. C., Sander, A. M. (2008). Perceptions of communication abilities for persons with traumatic brain injury: Validity of the La Trobe Communication Questionnaire. *Brain Inj.,* 22, 940–951

Weintraub, D. (2008). Dopamine and impulse control disorders in Parkinson’s disease. *Ann Neurol.,* 64(2):S93-100.

Biographical Sketches

Sara Palermo, PhD

Affiliation: Department of Psychology – University of Turin – Italy

Education:

- 2014 Ph.D. in Experimental Neuroscience
  Doctoral School in Life and Health Sciences – University of Turin
- 2009 M.Sc. in Clinical Psychology
  Department of Psychology – University of Turin

Address: Department of Psychology (Palazzo Badini), Via Verdi 10 (10124) Turin – Italy

Research and Professional Experience:

- For the Department of Psychology – University of Turin:
  2013-today Member of the research group "Neuropsychology of cognitive impairment and central nervous system degenerative diseases" (Research Area: Psychobiology and physiological psychology)
- For the Department of Neuroscience "Rita Levi Montalcini" – University of Turin:
  2014-today Member of the research group "Center for the Study of Movement Disorders" (Research Area: Neurology)
  2014-today Member of the research group "Placebo Responses Mapping" (Research Area: Physiology)

Professional Appointments:

- For the Department of Psychology – University of Turin:

2017-today	Post-Doc Research Fellow
2015-2016	Adjunct professor of the Psychophysiology-Lab
2014-today	Teaching assistant of the course "Neuropsychology of cognitive impairment and central nervous system degenerative diseases"
2014-today	Teaching assistant of the course "Forensic Neuropsychology"
2014-today	Teaching assistant of the course "Psychophysiology B"

- For the Department of Neuroscience "Rita Levi Montalcini" – University of Turin:

2014-2017	Post-Doc Research Fellow

Honors:

- Ordinary member of the Italian Society of Neuropsychology (SINP)
- Ordinary member of the Italian Association of Psychogeriatrics (AIP)

Publications Last 3 Years:

2017 Palermo S, Morese R, Zibetti M, Dematteis F, Sirgiovanni S, Stanziano M, Valentini MC, Lopiano L. Impulse control disorder and response-inhibition alterations in Parkinson's disease. A rare case of totally absent functionality of the medial-prefrontal cortex and review of literature. *J Adv Res*. 2017 Nov;8(6):713-716.

2017 Zibetti M, Palermo S, Vighetti S, Romagnolo A, Lopiano L. Deep brain stimulation influences on event-related potentials (P300) in Parkinson's disease. *Movement Disorders*, 32 (suppl 2): S137.

2017 S Palermo, R Morese, M Zibetti, F Dematteis, M ConsueloValentini, Lopiano L. Reduced GO/NOGO ACC-sensitive activity in a case of Parkinson's disease with impulse control disorders. *New Horizons in Clinical Case Reports* 1, 9

2017 Amanzio M, D'Agata F, Palermo S, Rubino E, Zucca M, Galati A, Pinessi L, Castellano G, Rainero I. Corrigendum to "Neural correlates of reduced awareness in instrumental activities of daily living in frontotemporal dementia" [*Exp. Gerontol.* 83 (2016) 158-164]. *Exp Gerontol.* pii: S0531-5565(17)30421-7.

2017 Palermo S. *Reduced self-awareness across pathologies: Involvement of the Anterior Cingulate Cortex.* Eds Nova Science Publishers, Hauppauge, NY. In: AA.VV. *Horizons in Neuroscience Research*, Volume 28. Chapter 3.

2017 Palermo S, Lopiano L, Zibetti M, Rosato R, Leotta D, Amanzio M. A novel framework for understanding reduced awareness of dyskinesias in Parkinson's Disease. *Parkinsonism and Related Disorders*, 39: 58-63

2017 Cauda F, Costa T, Nani A, Fava L, Palermo S, Bianco F, Duca S, Tatu K, Keller R. Are Schizophrenia, Autistic, and Obsessive Spectrum Disorders Dissociable on the Basis of Neuroimaging Morphological Findings? A Voxel-Based Meta-Analysis. *Autism Res*, 10(6): 1079-1095

2016 Amanzio M, Palermo S. Conceptualizing placebo as active component and adjunct in psychological treatment. Eds Oxford University Press, In: Sara Maltzman. Oxford *Handbook of Treatment Processes and Outcomes in Counseling Psychology*. Chapter 20.

2016 Amanzio M, Palermo S, Skyt I; Vase L. Lessons Learned from Nocebo Effects in Clinical Trials for Pain Conditions and Neurodegenerative Disorders. *Journal of Clinical Psychopharmacology*, 36(5): 475-482

2016 Amanzio M, D'Agata F, Palermo S, Rubino E, Zucca M, Galati A, Pinessi L, Castellano G, Rainero I. Neural correlates of reduced awareness in instrumental activities of daily living in frontotemporal dementia. *Exp Gerontol*, 83: 158-164

2016 Palermo S, Amanzio M, Zibetti M, Lopiano L. Dyskinesias-reduced-self-awareness and theory of mind in Parkinson's disease: A novel frame of interpretation. *Movement Disorders*, 31: S462-S462

2016 Palermo S, Lopiano L, Zibetti M, Morese R, Valentini MC, Amanzio M. Response-inhibition and Dyskinesias-Reduced-Self-Awareness in Parkinson's Disease: a piloting fMRI study. *Neuropsychological Trends*, 20: 134.

2016 Rainero I Amanzio M, D'Agata F, Galati A, Palermo S, Rubino E, Zucca M, Pinessi L, Castellano G. Frailty correlates with insula hypometabolism and frontal cortex atrophy in bvFTD. *Journal of Neurochemistry*, 138: 399-399

2016 Palermo S, Rainero R, Rubino E, Zucca M, Amanzio M. Frailty and cognitive decline. The role of metacognitive-executive dysfunction. *Journal of Alzheimer's Disease*, 53 (suppl1): S48-S48

2016 Rainero I Amanzio M, D'Agata F, Galati A, Palermo S, Rubino E, Zucca M, Pinessi L, Castellano G. Neural correlates of frailty in behavioral variant frontotemporal dementia. *Journal of Alzheimer's Disease*, 52 (suppl1): S23-S24.

2015 Palermo S, Benedetti F, Costa T, Amanzio M. Pain anticipation: An activation likelihood estimation meta-analysis of brain imaging studies. *Hum Brain Mapping*, 36 (5): 1648-61

2015 Palermo S, Cauda F, Costa T, Duca S, Gallino G, Geminiani G, Keller R, Amanzio M. Unawareness of Bipolar Disorder: The Role of the Cingulate Cortex. *Neurocase*, 21 (4): 438-47

2015 Cauda F, Costa T, Fava L, Palermo S, Bianco F, Duca S, Geminiani G, Tatu K, Keller R. *Predictability of autism, schizophrenic and obsessive spectra diagnosis. Toward a damage network approach.* bioRxiv, doi:

http://dx.doi.org/10.1101/014563
2015 Palermo S, Amanzio M, Zibetti M, Lopiano L.
Unawareness of dyskinesias in Parkinson's Disease: Is there a relationship with Theory of Mind dysfunctions?
Neurological Sciences, 36 (suppl29): S204

Rosalba Morese, PhD

Affiliations: Department of Psychology, University of Turin - Italy; Faculty of Communication Sciences, Università della Svizzera Italiana, Lugano – Switzerland

Education:

- 2015 Ph.D. in Neuroscience
  Doctoral School in Life and Health Sciences, University of Turin - Italy
- 2009 M.Sc. in Experimental Psychology
  Department of Psychology, University of Parma - Italy

Address: Via Po 14, 10123, Turin – Italy

Research and Professional Experience:

- For the Department of Psychology – University of Turin:
  2015-2017 Member of the research group "GIPSI - research Group on Inferential Processes in Social Interaction" (Research Area: Psychology - Neuroscience)
- For the Faculty of Communication Sciences – University of Lugano:
  2016-2017 Member of the research group "Psychology of Interpersonal Communication" (Research Area: Psychology - Neuroscience)

Professional Appointments:

- For the Department of Psychology – University of Turin:
  2015-2017 Post-Doc Research Fellow
  2015-2016 Adjunct professor of the General Psychology course
- For the Faculty of Communication Sciences – University of Lugano:
  2016-2017 Teaching assistant for the course of Social Psychology and Psychology of Communication

Publications Last 3 Years:

2017 Palermo S, Morese R, Zibetti M, Dematteis F, Sirgiovanni S, Stanziano M, Valentini MC, Lopiano L. Impulse control disorder and response-inhibition alterations in Parkinson's disease. A rare case of totally absent functionality of the medial-prefrontal cortex and review of literature. *J Adv Res*. 2017 Nov;8(6):713-716.

2017 Palermo S, Morese R, Zibetti M, Dematteis F, Valentini MC, Lopiano L. Reduced GO/NOGO ACC-sensitive activity in a case of Parkinson's disease with impulse control disorders. *New Horizons in Clinical Case Reports* 1, 9.

2017 Bosco FM, Parola A, Valentini MC, Morese R Neural correlates underlying the comprehension of deceitful and ironic communicative intentions. *Cortex*. 2017 Sep;94:73-86

2016 Rabellino, D, Morese* R, Ciaramidaro A, Bara BG, Bosco FM. Third-party punishment: altruistic and anti-social behaviours in in-group and out-group settings. *Journal of Cognitive Psychology*, 1-22. *corrisponding author.

2016 Palermo S, Lopiano L, Zibetti M, Morese R, Valentini MC, Amanzio M. Response-inhibition and Dyskinesias-Reduced-Self-Awareness 134 in Parkinson's Disease: a piloting fMRI study. In *Neuropsychological Trends*- ISSN:1970-321X

2016 Troni W, Boretto F, Di Sapio A, Melillo F, Morese R, Valentini MC. Simultaneous recording of motor related cortical potentials to different basal components of voluntary movements. *Clinical Neurophysiology*, 127(12), e327.

2016 Palermo S, Lopiano L, Zibetti M, Morese R, Valentini MC, Amanzio M. Response-inhibition and Dyskinesias-Reduced-Self-Awareness 134 in Parkinson's Disease: a piloting fMRI study. XXIV Congresso Nazionale della Società Italiana di Psicofisiologia. Milano, 27-29 Ottobre. In *Neuropsychological Trends*- ISSN:1970-321X.

2015 *Ear Acupuncture and fMRI. Akupunktur & Aurikulomedizin*. Romoli, M, Leobruni, S, Morese, R, Bosco, G, Valentini, C, 1:12-18. DOI: 10.1007/s15009-015-5316-1

2015 Morese R, Bosco FM, Lamm C, Valentini MC, Silani G. Social support modulates the neural correlates underlying social exclusion. In *Neuropsychological Trends*- ISSN:1970-321X.

In: Horizons in Neuroscience Research ISBN: 978-1-53613-286-1
Editors: A. Costa and E. Villalba

Chapter 6

NEURONAL LABELING OF THE RETINAL GANGLION CELLS: ADVANTAGES AND DISADVANTAGES OF LABELING WITH FLUORESCENT TRACERS

F. Germain[1,*], PhD, J. Vicente-Tejedor[1], PhD, C. Pérez-Rico[2], PhD and P. de la Villa[1], PhD

[1]Department of Biology of Systems,
Universidad de Alcalá, Madrid, Spain
[2]Department of Ophthalmology,
Hospital Príncipe de Asturias, Madrid, Spain

ABSTRACT

Background and objectives: The visual system is an approachable part of the central nervous system, which is suitable for investigating neuronal death, as well as to develop therapies toward its prevention. Mouse visual pathway has been used as a model to study degenerative

---

* Corresponding Author Email: francisco.germain@uah.es.

neurological disorders, especially after technology has allowed the generation of genetically engineered animals. To make an accurately cell quantification of retinal ganglion cells (RGCs) is one of the main objectives in these works, due to its high variability among diverse strains of mice. The goal of this study was to compare two types of retrograde axonal transport in RGCs.

Material and methods: After anaesthetizing the mouse, the midline of skin, on the top of head, was cut, and small holes were made in the skull following stereotactic localization of *superior colliculi*. Following withdrawal of a tiny portion of bone, part of the cerebral cortex was aspirated and the *superior colliculi* were exposed, placing a sponge soaked in the retrograde tracer Fluorogold on its surface. One week later, under anesthesia, after cutting the left superior rectus and left superior oblique eye muscles, the optic nerve was dorsally exposed and cut. Then, a piece of spongostan soaked in dextran tetramethyl rhodamine (DTMR) was applied on the optic nerve stump to label RGCs. At different post-labeling times, eyes were enucleated and the retinas fixed and mounted to study. Left retinas (injured) were analyzed with both labeling, FG and DTMR; while right retinas (uninjured) were only observed under FG labeling.

Results and discussion: Different tracers stained RGCs in a different way. FG-labeled RGCs had a typical bright punctate and diffuse blue fluorescence, delineating their soma and the initial portion of their primary dendrites; while DTMR labeled cells had a red bright fluorescence. Counts of DTMR labeling cells were less numerous than FG labeling cells. Probably, it was due to a problem in axonal transport after injury. Also, some RGCs were labeled only with DTMR. It could be explained because there is a minority of RGCs that project to other nuclei different to *superior colliculi.* After optic nerve injury, a progressive decrease in RGCs number and an increase in microglial cells number were observed. When labeled RGCs are phagocytosed by microglial cells, tracer was incorporated into the microglial cell and become fluorescent.

Conclusion: Different tracers and different places to apply along the visual pathways must be considered depending on the specific characteristics required by the project being carried out.

1. INTRODUCTION

The optic pathway is an approachable part of the brain, which is suitable for investigating different injury-induced neuronal death [1, 2, 3], as well as to develop therapies toward its prevention [4, 5, 6].

Within the visual pathway, the retina is an optimal tissue for the study of neuronal damage due to its easy access and orderly structure. Specifically, retinal ganglion cells (RGC) have been chosen frequently to perform such studies. The models of retinal diseases with affection of the optic nerve allow us to know how and why RGC die. Thereby, to know the mechanisms of cellular degeneration opens the way to essay new therapies through genetic manipulation.

1.1. Visual Pathway and Relay Nuclei

The visual pathway is composed of a set of interconnected structures that make visual perception possible. Light information is collected by retinal photoreceptors and processed within the retina and further structures. Anatomically, the optic pathway consists of retina, optic nerve, optic chiasm, optic tract, lateral geniculate nucleus (LGN), *superior colliculi (*SCi), optic tracts, and visual cortex (see Figures 1 and 2).

The axons of the RGC on leaving the eyeball form the optic nerve (II cranial nerve). The optic nerve fibers on the medial sides of each retina cross over (decussate) to the opposite hemisphere at the optic chiasm (decussation of nasal fibers). In humans and primates, 50% of all optical axons cross the midline in this area, so that the fibers of the nasal hemi-retina are crossed, while the fibers of the temporal hemi-retina are maintained ipsilaterally. The proportion of fibers that cross midline changes with the specie. Unlike in humans, in mice and rats, the percentage of RGC that is ipsilaterally projected is approximately 2.6% and 5%, respectively, so about 95-97% cross midline [7, 8, 9, 10]. After chiasm, the fibers of the ipsilateral temporal retina and the contralateral nasal retina of each side are brought together to form the optical tracts, therefore each cerebral hemisphere lead the information coming from the contralateral visual hemi-world. Subsequently, the optic tracts project to three main subcortical areas: *superior colliculi* (or tectum), which forms part of the quadrigeminal tubercle; mesencephalic pretectum; and lateral geniculate nucleus of the thalamus. In addition to these three subcortical structures, the optic tracts also project to the suprachiasmatic nuclei, the pregeniculate and the nuclei that make up the accessory visual system. Slices of these nuclei are shown in Figure 2. Approximately 90% of retinal axons make synaptic contact in LGN (see Figure 1). This nucleus is considered the most important relay station in transporting visual information to the cerebral cortex.

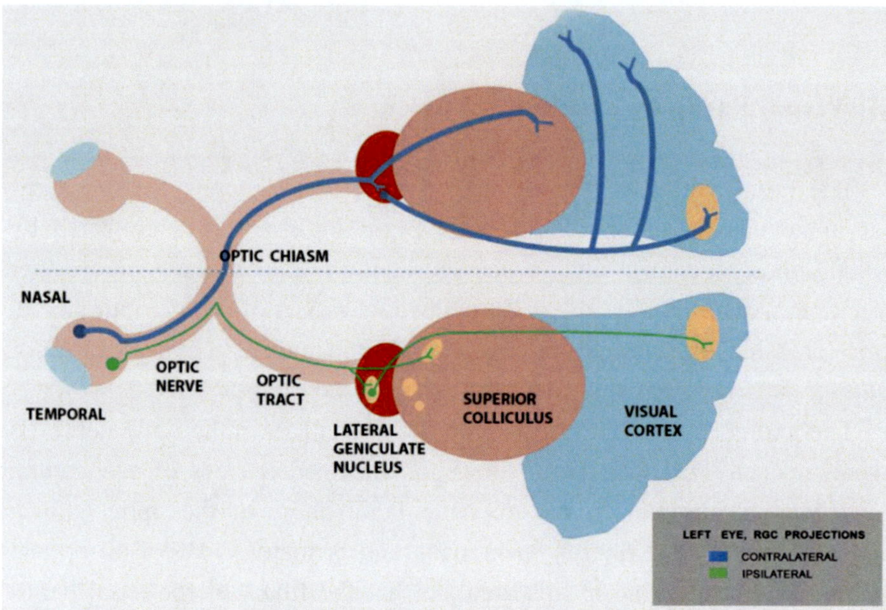

Figure 1. Visual pathway in mouse. Visual pathway begins in each eye. Retinal ganglion cells project, ipsi and contralateral, their axons to lateral geniculate nucleus and *superior colliculus* to make synaptic contact in different relay nucleus, and beyond with visual cortex.

The central visual system follows a general organization called retinotopy, that is, neighboring cells in the retina feed information to neighboring places in their target structures, the LGN, *superior colliculi*, and striate cortex. The two-dimensional representation of the visual world is mapped onto the two-dimensional surface of the retina and is repeated on the subsequent structures of the visual system [11]. Retinotopic maps, also called visual field maps, are a type of topographic organization. Many brain structures that respond to visual input, such as much of the visual

cortex, visual nuclei of the brain stem (*superior colliculi*), and thalamus (lateral geniculate nucleus and the pulvinar) follow this organization. Specifically, in the LGN, there are several layers responsible for processing separately different aspects of vision (movement, shape and color). In each of such layers, the visual field is organized in a retinotopic way. In addition, due to the segregation of axons after the optic chiasm, each LGN has a retinotopic representation of the contralateral half of the visual field.

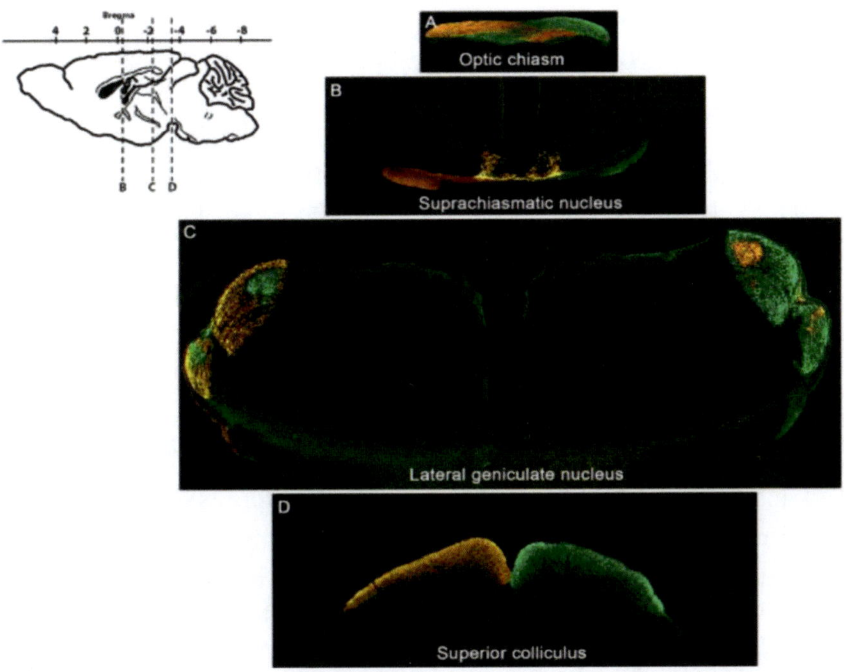

Figure 2. Different levels of visual pathway after labeling with intraocular injection of cholero toxin. A, Labeled slice at the level of optic chiasm. B, Labeled slice at the level of suprachiasmatic nucleus (-0.34 mm from Bregma). C, Labeled slice at the level of lateral geniculate nucleus (-2.18 mm from Bregma). Labeling in red corresponds to left eye and labeling in green corresponds to right eye. D, Labeled slice at the level of *superior colliculus* (-3.52 mm from Bregma). Optic pathway was labeling with cholero toxin (CTX 488 (Cy2 -green) in the right eye and CTX 555 (Cy3 -red) in the left eye). It is possible to appreciate how optic nerve fibers change to the other hemisphere in the optic chiasm.

From the LGN, after making synaptic contact, axons are sent to form the optical radiations and reach the primary visual cortex, which is located in the middle surface of the posterior poles of the cerebral hemispheres. Subsequently, the information collected in the primary visual cortex is sent to multiple centers outside such cortex and dedicated to visual processing (perception of movement, depth, shape, and color).

In rodent visual pathway, the axons leave the optic papilla retinotopically organized [12, 13, 14, 15, 16, 17, 18]. Rodent RGCs project to the following regions of the brain: suprachiasmatic nucleus, accessory optic nucleus, pretectal nucleus, ventrolateral geniculate nucleus, dorsal lateral geniculate nucleus (DLGN), and superior colliculus, being this last one the main projection zone of RGCs [19, 20, 21, 8, 9]. The SCi are two protuberances located in the dorsal part of the midbrain, rostral to the *inferior colliculi* and composed of superficial and deeper layers. Superficial or visual layers are: *Stratum Zonale, Stratum Griseum Superficiale, Stratum Opticum* (its function consist on receiving retinal afferents and process the visual stimuli). Deeper layers are: intermediate gray layer *(Stratum Griseum Intermediale),* intermediate white layer *(Stratum Album Intermediale),* deep gray layer *(Stratum Griseum Profundum)* and deep white layer *(Stratum Album Profundum),* responsible for processing auditory and somatosensory information. The axons of the RGC reach the *Stratum Opticum*, branch out, and form synaptic terminals that terminate mainly in the superficial gray layer *(Stratum Griseum)* and the zonal layer (*Stratum Zonale).* See these layers of *superior colliculi* in Figure 3. All the distribution of RGC axons in the SCi follows a determined topography, so that the axons coming from the nasal retina project to the caudal half of the SCi, those from the temporal retina to the rostral half, those of the retina superior to the lateral side of SCi, and those of the inferior retina to the medial part of SCi [22, 23]. In rodents, the visual information that reaches the cerebral cortex related to visual image formation also comes from the lateral geniculate nuclei, but the *superior colliculi* is the main retino-recipient subcortical nucleus.

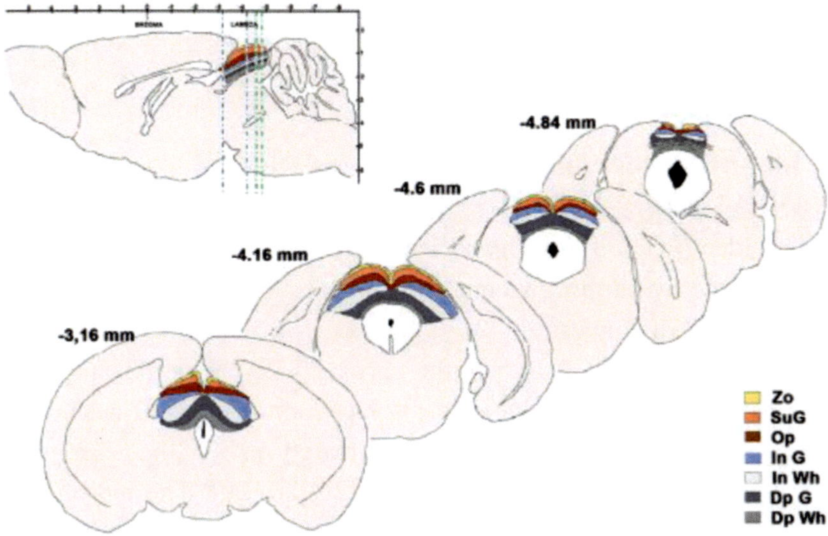

Figure 3. Sections of *superior colliculus*. In the left corner, a medial sagittal view of mouse brain is scaled. Four lines crossing *superior colliculus* point different slides, which are viewed below. Surgical approach was done between the first two lines (blue). *Superior colliculus* sub-layers are represented in different colors: Zo, zonal layer; Su G, superficial gray layer; Op, optic nerve of the *superior colliculus*; In G, intermediate gray layer; InWh, intermediate white layer; DpG, Deep gray; DpWh, deep white layer.

Mouse RGCs projects to several nuclei like the suprachiasmatic, the accessory optic, the pretectal, the ventral lateral geniculate, the dorsal lateral geniculate, and the SCi [24]. It has been reported that most RGCs projections have the *superior colliculi* (SCi) (Figure 2 and 3A) as important target [19, 20, 8] and expand their processes following a very accurately way [21, 22, 23, 9]. Given the variability between species, in any studied model it is necessary to know the number of RGCs that project to SCi [8].

Mouse visual pathway has been widely used as a model to analyze morphological and functional characteristics of degenerative neurological disorders. The development of technology has allowed the generation of genetically engineered animals, and consequently the use of this model has increased. However, the numbers of RGCs are highly variable among diverse strains of mice [25, 8]. This is the reason to make an accurately cell quantification previously to any functional or morphological RGC study.

1.2. Identification and Quantification of RGC

The identification and quantification of RGC are vital to know the effects caused by harmful agents, as well as to assess the effectiveness of neuroprotective therapies.

It is known that RGC are not the only cells that form the ganglion cell layer of the rodent retina, since the displaced amacrine cells are in similar proportion [26, 20, 27]. In mouse, approximately 59% of the neurons of the RGC layer are displaced amacrine cells [26, 28, 29]. The morphological criteria show that displaced amacrine cells and small RGC have a similar size, so this criterion does not serve to distinguish this class of retinal neurons [1, 30].

Mammal retinal ganglion cells population are distributed in a central-peripheral gradient, showing the highest density in the superior retina in mice [26, 31, 8] in rats [32, 31, 9] and in other rodents.

1.3. Techniques Used for Labeling RGC

1.3.1. Immunodetection

Along with neuronal tracers, immunohistochemistry is the most used method since it allows the unequivocal identification of RGC. Such identification is possible by using a reliable marker. The protein used as a marker must satisfy two requirements: to be specifically expressed by most of RGCs [33, 34] and that after a lesion the RGC loss correlates with the death of cells (expression level of the marker).

The use of antibodies against Thy-1, a protein that is selectively expressed in RGCs [35, 36] has been used to identify RGC. However, the lack of correlation between the decrease in the expression of this protein in injured CGR and its death make this method unsuitable for determining cell survival [37]. In addition, in cell injury models, such as the optic nerve section, it has been observed its expression in the retinal Müller cells, so it is not specific of RGC [34].

Immunodetection of BEX ½ recognizes the cell bodies of the RGCs and their projections, so it is a suitable marker for the study of the cellular morphological changes associated with the lesion. However, due to its axonal expression is not an appropriate marker for quantitative analysis. Similarly occurs with the detection of synuclein mRNA in RGCs, which was developed to specifically label RGC [38]. However, this protein is expressed in neuronal body, axons, and dendrites of RGCs, making automatic quantification difficult.

The Brn3 family is composed by three transcription factors (Brn3a/*Pou4f1*, Brn3b/*Pou4f2*, Brn3c/*Pou4f3*) [39] that are expressed by different sets of neurons of the retina [40, 10]. Brn3b is very important for RGC differentiation, survival and axon pathfinding [41], Brn3c is required for ipsilateral projections [2] and Brn3a participates in the regulation of RGC dendritic stratification [42].

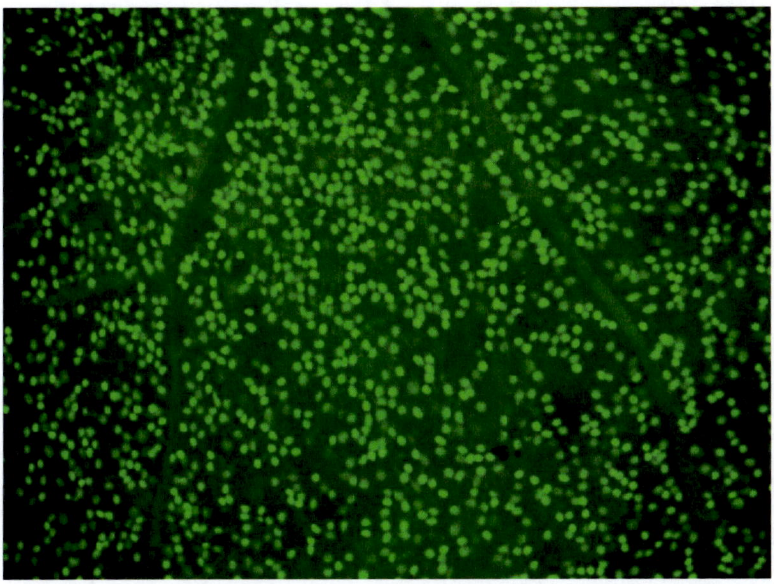

Figure 4. Mouse retinal ganglion cells immunolabeled with Brn3a antibody.

Both mouse and rat express Brn3a in a vast majority RGC population [43, 44]. This Brn3a expression is maintained in those alive RGCs after being injured [45]. These two reasons make Brn3a immunodetection a very good tool to quantify RGC in these species [10]. Mouse Brn3a expression is shown in Figure 4.

1.3.2. Labeling by Fluorescent Molecules

Other strategies used to stain visual pathway are based on placing fluorescent molecules in different sites along the pathway. Then, such fluorochromes are retrogradely transported through axonal RGC towards their somas to be stored within, and causing a brilliant labeling.

1.3.2.1. Types of Fluorochromes

These substances are named tracers. The persistence of this fluorescence indicates that membranes perform their function and cell is healthy [46]. There are numerous tracers that have been successfully used for labeling neurons like Fast-blue [47, 48, 49]; DiI [47], that is a fluorescent lipophilic cationic indocarbocyanine dye usually made as a perchlorate salt and retained in the lipid bilayers; DiAsp [50] or 4Di-10ASP (4-(4-(Dicecylamino)styryl)-N-Methylpyridinium Iodide) [51], molecule that contains a C10 alkyl chain to be inserted into membranes, in that moment its fluorophore parallel shows a strong fluorescence; FluoroGold (2-hidroxiestilbeno 4,4'dicarboxamidinebis (metanosulfonato)) [9] or its equivalent hydroxystilbamidine methanesulfonate (OHSt) [52, 53]; or dextrantetramethylrhodamine (DTMR) [9, 53].

1.3.2.2. Places to Apply the Tracers

1.3.2.2.1. Into the Eye

By using these tracers both optic pathways may be labeled differently, which is useful to assess individually both visual pathways after a unilateral injury. This method consists in inject cholera toxins (CTX) into the eye, such substances have a different chromophore added for each eye (CTX 488, Cy2 –green and CTX 555, Cy3 –red) (see Figure 2). After intraocular injection, CTX goes into the RGC and stains their axons to reach the optic chiasm (OC) (see Figure 2A) through the optic nerve, where they cross to the other side (decussation). In slices, made at this level of the optic pathway, the origin of the fibers can be distinguished as a function of color. The decussation of the fibers from both eyes subsequently determines the contralateral marking of both suprachiasmatic nuclei (see Figure 2B). Through the optic tracts CTX labeling reaches the lateral geniculate nucleus (see Figure 2C). From there, axonal projections reach the *superior colliculus* (see Figure 2D). In these projection nuclei, thanks to the use of CTX that mark in red and green depending on the eye, it is possible to distinguish the ipsilateral and contralateral regions. An injury that affects only one eye would cause a deficit in labeling the ipsi and contralateral projection nuclei of that eye.

1.3.2.2.2. On the Superior Colliculus

One of most used places to label RGC in rodents is the projection targets of RGC, such as *superior colliculus* [54, 55, 56, 57, 53], which is the main projection territory of the RGC [20] and therefore identifies practically all RGC in rodents.

1.3.2.2.3. Into the Optic Nerve

There are other sites along visual pathways for labeling RGCs, like the optic nerve (ON), intracraneally [30] or intraorbitally [30, 53]. It has the advantage that includes all the axons that emerge from the RGC, not only those that go to SCi. Other studies have reported that RGC could be labeled by ON injection of tracers in larger species, like rabbit [48, 49]. However, in mouse it is very difficult to inject any substance into the optic nerve without causing any damage. Alternatively, it is possible to cut the optic nerve and labeling the stump [47, 53], although in this case the retinal damage caused must be accounted.

It has been mentioned that a degenerative process could alter the cellular expression of proteins, which would imply the inability of the immunohistochemistry to detect them. In order to ensure that this possible expression deficit does not affect the RGC visualization, other methods such as fluorescent tracers are often used. Below we show in detail two techniques based on using fluorescent tracers that avoid such problems.

2. RGC Double Labeling from the Optic Nerve and Its Projection Nucleus (Superior Colliculus) in Mouse

2.1. Methods

2.1.1. Animals

All experimental procedures were carried out in accordance with the European Union statement for the use of laboratory animals (Directive 86/609/CEE). Two-month old, wild-type mice (Charles River Laboratories), weighing 20–30 g, were used in these studies. Animals were reared in an artificial 12-h light/dark cycle with food and water *ad libitum*. Illumination was 30 cd/m^2.

2.1.2. Surgical Techniques

2.1.2.1. Surgical Procedures and Retrograde Labeling of RGCs from *Superior Colliculi*

Mice were anaesthetized with an intraperitoneal injection of saline solution (NaCl 0.9%), containing ketamine (70 mg/kg; Ketalar, Parke-Davis, Wellington, New Zealand) and xylazine (7 mg/kg; Rompun, Bayer, Leverkusen, Germany). For comparison, RGCs were labeled with the retrograde tracers Fluorogold (FG) (2-hydroxystilbene-4,4′-dicarboxamidine bis [methasulfonate]) (Sigma) or its equivalent hydroxystilbamidine methanesulfonate (OHSt) (Molecular Probes, Leiden, The Netherlands) with similar fluorescent and tracer properties to fluorogold [52, 8, 9]; and dextrantetramethylrhodamine (DTMR) (Molecular Probes, Eugene, OR, USA) was applied on the optic nerve stump. FG was applied to both SCi and DTMR just on the cut ON.

After shaving the top of head, a sagittal incision in the midline of skin was made. The edges of the incision were separated and small holes were made with a drill bit at an area on either side of the midline, such as Figure 5B shows (blue lines). To make a stereotactic localization of SCi (labeled in red color in Figure 5B), the mouse brain atlas by Paxinos and Franklin was used [58].

The holes were perforated close to midline, from 2 mm anterior to lambda until almost lambda point (see Figure 5B). The hole reaches laterally up to 1.5 mm. Such action was carried out with great care not to drill the mid-sagittal or lamboids sutures, because a venous sinus sits beneath and could cause bleeding.

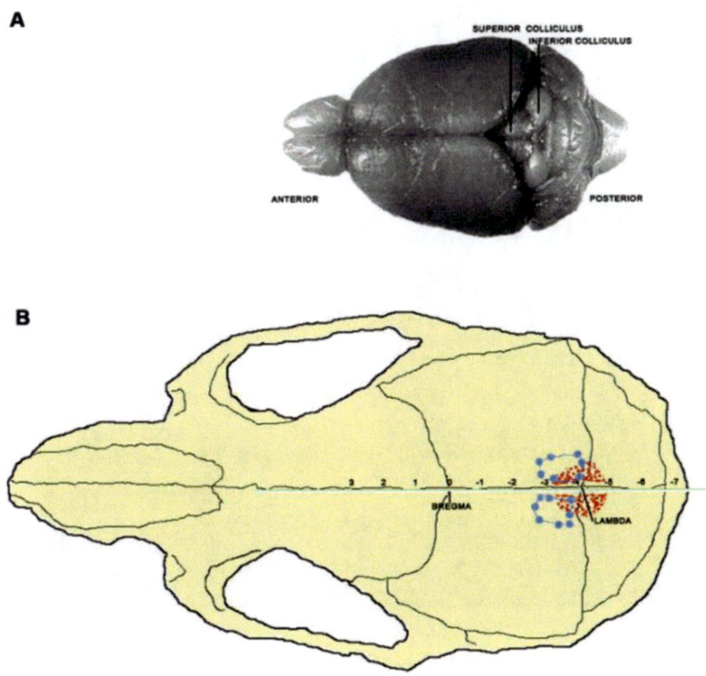

Figure 5. Location of *superior colliculus*. Dorsal view of mouse brain (A). Dorsal view of mouse skull (B). In B, *superior colliculus* is labeled in red and surgical approach in blue. Blue dots show the locations where holes were made in the skull. Finally, in each hemisphere, new holes were made following the blue line until the piece of bone was pull up to allow access to brain.

After removing that portion of skull, cerebral cortex was exposed (see Figure 6A). With a pump of suction, a part of granular and agranular cortex, just above SCi, was withdrawn (See Figure 3), and the anterior part of SCi was left visible. It was recognized because white color (see Figure 6A) changes to reddish (see Figure 6B).

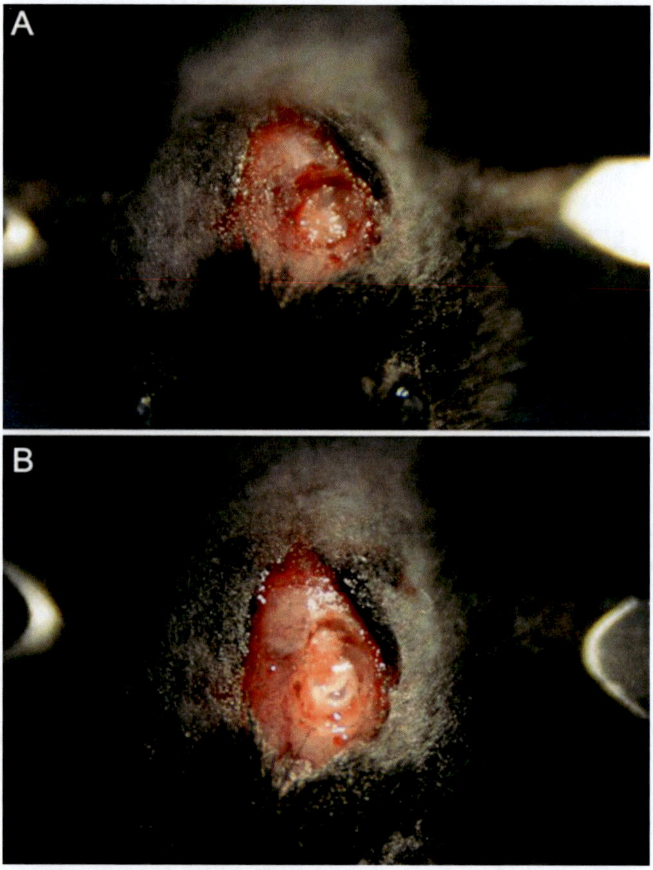

Figure 6. Surgical approaching to *superior colliculus*.

After pulled the piece of bone up, the white cortex is visible (A). After vacuuming the outer part of cortex with care and slowly, the surface changed its color from white to pink showing the *superior colliculus* (B).

A small pledget of gelatine sponge (Espongostan Film, Ferrosan A/S, Søborg, Denmark), soaked in saline solution containing 3% FG

(Fluorochrome Inc., Engelwood, CO, USA) and 10% dimethyl sulphoxide (DMSO), was applied over the entire surface of the Sci. Different phases of labeling have been shown in the figures. Previous studies in control mice have reported that FG application to both SCi, which are the main retino-recipient target regions in the brain, results 1 week later in the labeling of approximately 96.6% of the RGCs population in C57BL/6 adult mice. This method was based on other previously described [47, 59, 8]. Finally, the skin wound was closed with several stitches.

2.1.2.2. Optic Nerve Transection

One week after labeling SCi, the left optic nerve was intraorbitally transected and RGCs labeled from the stump with another distinct molecule.

Both eyelids were kept wide open through fixation with adhesive tape to the supporting base. The capsule of Tenon was dissected at the scleral-corneal edge in the whole upper half of the eye. After superior and oblique eye muscles were cut, adhesions of the eyeball were separated until posterior pole using scissors (by opening) or an ocular absorbing sponge, being careful not to injure any blood vessel.

The eye was displaced outside the orbit to expose the dorsal side of the optic nerve. In this way, meningeal sheaths surrounding optic nerve could be opened and the nerve completely cut near the eye cup (2 mm behind the eyecup). Care was taken not to injure blood vessels, especially the ophthalmic artery that enters the sclera from the ventral margin of the optic nerve [60]. This was the main reason to cut optic nerve from the dorsal side.

After axotomy, RGCs were retrogradely labeled by applying a piece of spongostan soaked in 0.1% DTMR at the optic nerve stump.

Following surgery, an antibiotic solution containing polymyxin B, neomycin, and gramicidin (Oftalmowell, Medeva Pharma, Madrid, Spain) was applied to the orbital space and the wound of eyelids sutured. Finally, a solution of 2% Methocel (Ciba Vision AG, 8442 Hetlingen, Switzerland) was applied on the cornea to prevent ocular desiccation.

2.1.3. Tissue Preparation

Animals were killed with an overdose of sodium pentobarbital. To maintain retinal orientation, a signal was made on the superior pole of each eye with a hot needle, previously to enucleating. A cut was made on cornea surface with a scalpel to allow fixation solution to penetrate into the eye. This solution is composed by 4% para-formaldehyde in mol/L phosphate buffer (pH 7.4) for 1 h at room temperature. Then, the retina was dissected out from the eyecup, flat-mounted vitreous side up. Four cuts were carried out on retina to show four areas, like four petals of a flower. Left retinas (injured) were studied with both labeling, FG and DTMR; while right retinas (uninjured) were only observed under FG labeling.

2.1.4. Quantification of RGC Population in Rodents

The quantification of RGCs, once identified, can be performed by automatic or manual methods. To quantify RGC, pictures showing a standard retinal area size (214 x 161 mm^2) were taken. This size was chosen because it allows to distinguish RGC from other cells. Any cell with a rounded soma and a diameter exceeding 8 μm was regarded as a RGC [61, 62, 63]. Cell counting could be performed in control and injured retinas at different times after optic nerve section (ONS). All cell counts were performed in a blind fashion by the same investigator.

The most used methods are:

- **Indirect quantification of RGC**. It is accepted that optic nerve is formed by the axons of the RGC, so that each axon would correspond to a RGC, by counting the axons of the ON the number of RGCs could be estimated. Estimates made in rat indicate that the number of RGCs of the adult rat retina ranges between 96,200 and 118,300 [64, 65]. In mouse, the number of axons quantified is 64,746 [66].
- **Manual RGC quantification**. This method is performed by selecting several counting areas (in the dorsal, ventral, lateral, and medial areas) in flat mounted whole retina, in which the calculation of the average cell density is performed after manual

counting of immuno-stained RGCs [1, 30, 55, 67]. Four pictures in the central retina, 0.5 mm away from the optic disc; and four in the peripheral retina, more than 1 mm away from the optic disc.

- **Automatic identification of RGC.** Through the automatic analysis of the whole retina the pattern of distribution of RGC can be known (maps of cellular isodensity) and estimate the total number of RGC. The cell density is automatically quantified by areas of interest and its data are transported to a computer program for its graphical representation (SigmaPlot® 9.0 for Windows®, *Systat Software, Inc.*, Richmond, CA) through the construction of isodensity maps. Thereby, cells can be counted after staining with neuronal tracers (fluorogold or OHSt (hydroxystilbamidine methanesulfonate)) or immunolabeling with Brn3a [68].

3. Results

3.1. RGC Labeling

The objective of this study was to compare two types of RGC labeling by retrograde axonal transport with respect to other types of methods. Retinal ganglion cells can be retrograde labeled by fluorescent tracers placed in different locations along the visual pathway. Those remaining fluorescent cells after injury are still alive [46].

Labeling properties depend on the fluorochrome used. In addition, the same tracer may cause light differences in intensity labeling. These differences were maximal with DTMR. Alternatively, FG-labeled RGC had a typical bright punctate and diffuse blue fluorescence delineating their soma, and sometimes the initial portion of their primary dendrites (Figure 7, 7A labeled with Fluorogold and 7B with DTMR). These cells were disposed in a regular distribution throughout the RGC layer, although some scattered cells were also found in the inner nuclear layer.

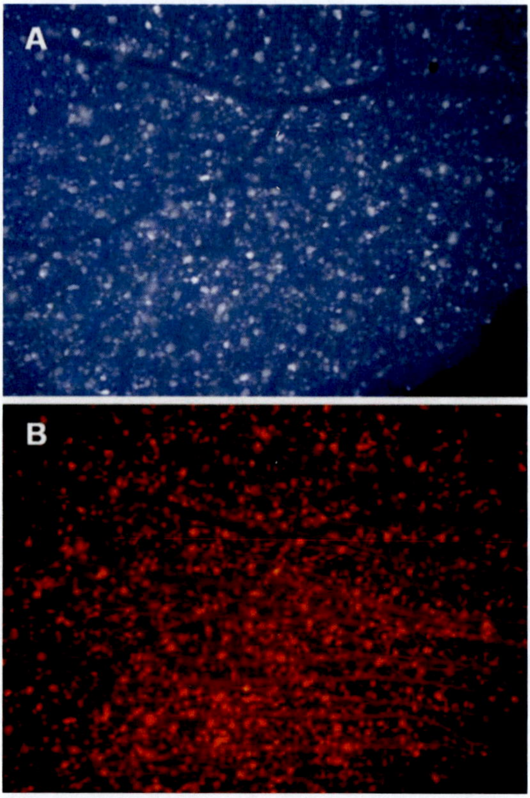

Figure 7. Mouse retinal ganglion cells in control retinas.

RGCs viewed after labeling with fluorogold from *superior colliculus* (A) and DTMR from optic nerve stump (B). The surgery to label with fluorogold was carried out 7 days before, axotomy and DTMR labeling was carried out 2 days before the sacrifice.

After optic nerve injury, two kinds of processes could be observed. A progressive decrease in RGC number and an increase in microglial cells number (pointed by the red arrow in Figure 8A). When labeled RGC are phagocytosed by microglial cells, the tracer is incorporated into the microglial cell and become fluorescent [69].

To count RGC it is necessary to distinguish both types of cells using morphological criteria. Microglial cells are smaller and spiculated (see several examples in Figure 8, 8A labeled with Fluorogold and 8B with DTMR).

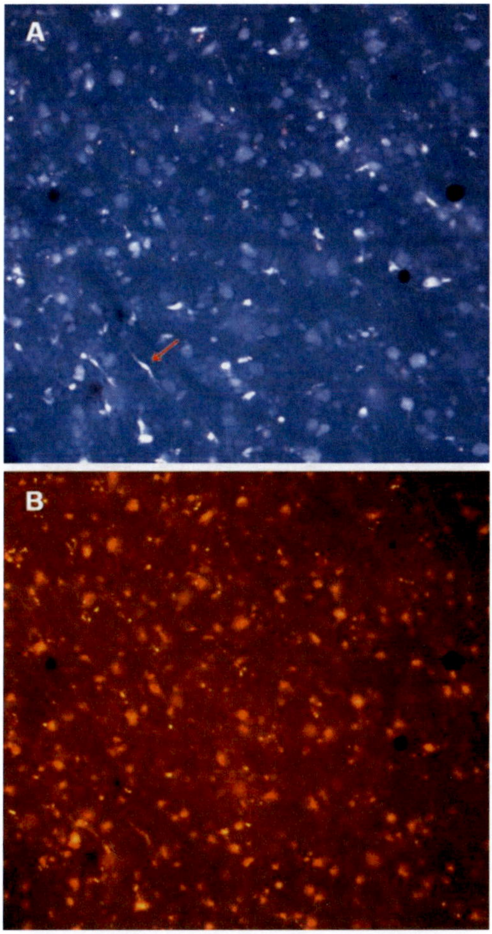

Figure 8. Mouse retinal ganglion cells 7 days after axotomy.

Some days after axotomy, in addition to RGC, it is possible to see some microglial cells labeled by tracers (red arrow). Microglia is visible with both fluorescent tracers.

3.2. RGCs Count

Retinal FG-labeled cells could be counted one week after staining SCi. This is the time taken by tracer to reach retina from SCi. However, after optic nerve section (DTMR-labeling) RGCs count should be done as soon as possible because RGC begin to die. This time point is estimated in 2 days, minimal time to reach somas from optic nerve stump [47], and surviving cells are not significant decreased yet, as we confirmed with FG-labeling and it is reported in the literature [43].

The appearance of DTMR-labeled RGCs (axotomized cells) in the first four days was similar to control FG-labeled RGC (Figure 7). However, in the following days some differences were observed respect to healthy retinas [53]. Fluorescence becomes brighter and more punctate, especially in DTMR-labeled RGC.

When these retinas were examined for doubly labeled RGC, it was found that not all DTMR-labeled RGC were labeled with FG and vice versa. There were also some FG-labeled RGC that were not labeled with DTMR. Because FG was applied to the SCi and DTMR was applied to the ON, it is possible that RGC labeled only with DTMR represent a small population of RGC that do not project to the SCi [70, 19, 21]. Likewise, RGC just FG labeled represent the fraction of RGC population that, due to problems in axonal transport, were not marked with DTMR after placing it in the stump. Count of DTMR-labeled RGC showed a significant fewer number of cells than FG-labeled RGC. This implies that axonal transport was damaged, but allowed a significant labeling of RGC.

Both, fluorescent tracers and Brn3a immunodetection, have their advantages and disadvantages. The FG tracer informs us that the RGC maintain their retrograde axonal transport active, since it is actively transported. However, as an inconvenient, some days after ON injury, microglia cells appear fluorescent in the retina. This labeling occurs because the cells of the microglia phagocytose the stained and died RGCs, and the tracer is accumulated in the phagosomes of microglia, so that they are also "labeled." This process is known as trans-cellular labeling [71, 72]. Although the number of RGC can be counted manually, since they are morphologically distinct from microglia cells, such transcellular labeling make the automatic counting of RGC be inaccurate.

The detection of RGC using immunohistofluorescent techniques has certain advantages over the use of tracers, since it does not require surgical manipulations and microglia cells are not labeled during the evolution of the study.

However, Brn3a immunodetection does not inform about axonal transport, since Brn3a is an endogenous protein that stops being expressed in RGCs when these cells undergo apoptosis. Thus, Brn3a immunodetection allows a more realistic temporal course of death [10, 44], since it identifies, quantifies and evaluates the loss of RGC in the adult mouse *"ex vivo."* The combined use of both methods has allowed, for example, to describe that in models of ocular hypertension there is firstly a loss of axonal transport, followed by death of RGC [68].

CONCLUSION

In conclusion there are several advantages and disadvantages for these methods:

Tracers

Advantages: It labels the cells and tells us about the axonal transport, regardless of whether certain proteins are expressed or not, so it is not necessary to find specific antibodies. Following tracer injection into the ON it is possible to label all the RGC axons that leave outside the eye. The transcellular labeling of the microglia can be an advantage when these cells are the specific aim of study.

Disadvantages:

a) Due to surgery: previous experience is necessary, hemorrhages (intracranial or intraorbital venous sinuses, depending on the type), waiting time for the tracer to reach the RGC, elimination of excessive amount of cerebral cortex.

b) Due to place of labeling:

i. In the SCi, it only labels those RGC that project in it, so that it is necessary to know that percentage in each species.

ii. In the optic nerve, when RGC are stained after ON section, such injury initiates the apoptosis of the RGC. It is possible to avoid this problem by just pricking into the optic nerve.

c) Transcellular labeling of the microglia makes it difficult to count RGC

Immunodetection

Advantages: Surgical manipulation is not necessary, avoiding all the inconveniences that it entails. No transcellular labeling of the microglia occurs. It allows to label simultaneously several different cells or proteins, so that studies of cellular or structural relations can be made.

Disadvantages: the loss of protein expression may prevent the labeling

Acknowledgment

The authors thanks to Mrs. Gemma Fernández for her English corrections.

References

[1] Villegas-Pérez, M. P., Vidal-Sanz, M., Bray G. M., Aguayo, A. J. (1988). Influences of peripheral nerve grafts on the survival and regrowth of axotomized retinal ganglion cells in adult rats. *Journal of Neuroscience, 8,* 265–280.

[2] Wang, S. W., Mu, X., Bowers, W. J., Kim, D. S., Plas, D. J., et al. (2002). Brn3b/Brn3c double knockout mice reveal an unsuspected role for Brn3c in retinal ganglion cell axon outgrowth. *Development, 129,* 467–477.

[3] Agudo, M., Pérez-Marín, M. C., Lönngren, U., Sobrado, P., Conesa, A., Cánovas, I. et al. (2008). Time course profiling of the retinal transcriptome after optic nerve transection and optic nerve crush. *Molecular Vision, 14,* 1050–1063.

[4] Vidal-Sanz, M., Lafuente, M., Sobrado-Calvo, P., Sellés-Navarro, I., Rodríguez, E., Mayor-Torroglosa, S. et al. (2000). Death and neuroprotection of retinal ganglion cells after different types of injury. *Neurotoxicity Research, 2,* 215–227.

[5] Avilés-Trigueros, M., Mayor-Torroglosa, S., García-Avilés, A., Lafuente, M. P., Rodríguez, M. E., Miralles de Imperial, J. et al. (2003). Transient ischemia of the retina results in massive degeneration of the retinotectal projection: Longterm neuroprotection with brimonidine. *Experimental Neurology, 184,* 767–777.

[6] Mayor-Torroglosa, S., De la Villa, P., Rodríguez, M. E., López-Herrera, M. P., Avilés-Trigueros, M., García-Avilés, A., et al. (2005). Ischemia results 3 months later in altered ERG, degeneration of inner layers, and deafferented tectum: Neuroprotection with brimonidine. *Investigative Ophthalmology Visual Science, 46,* 3825–3835.

[7] Métin, C., Irons, W. A., Frost, D. O. (1995). Retinal ganglion cells in normal hamsters and hamsters with novel retina projections. I Number, distribution and size. *J Comp Neurol., 353*, 179-199.

[8] Salinas-Navarro, M., Jiménez-López, M., Valiente-Soriano, F. J. et al. (2009a). Retinal ganglion cell population in adult albino and pigmented mice: a computerized analysis of the entire population and its spatial distribution. *Vision Research, 49,* 637–647.

[9] Salinas-Navarro, M., Mayor-Torroglosa, S., Jiménez-López, M., Avilés-Trigueros, M., Holmes, T., Lund, R. D., et al. (2009b). A computerized analysis of the entire retinal ganglion cell population and its spatial distribution in adult rats. *Vision Research, 49,* 115–126.

[10] Nadal-Nicolás, F. M., Jiménez-López, M., Salinas-Navarro, M., Sobrado-Calvo, P., Alburquerque-Béjar, J. J., Vidal-Sanz, M., Agudo-Barriuso, M. (2012). Whole number, distribution and co-expression of brn3 transcription factors in retinal ganglion cells of

adult albino and pigmented rats. *PLoS One., 7:e49830. Epub 2012 Nov 16.*

[11] Bear, M. F., Connors, B. W., Paradiso, M. A. (2008). *Neuroscience exploring the brain, 3th edition*. Lippincott, Williams and Wilkins. Editor Susan Katz. Baltimore, USA.

[12] Guillery, R. W., Mason, C. A., Taylor, J. S. (1995). Developmental determinants at the mammalian iptic chiasm *J Neurosci., 15,* 4727-4737.

[13] Fitzgibbon, T., Reese, B. E. (1996). Organization of reinal ganglion cell axons in the optic fiber layer and nerve of fetal ferrets. *Vis Neurosci., 13,* 847-861.

[14] Jeffery, G. (2001). Architecture of the optic chiasm and the mechanisms that sculpt its development. *Physiol Rev., 81*, 1393-1414.

[15] Jeffery, G., Levitt, J. B., Cooper, H. M. (2008). Segregated hemispheric pathways through the optic chiasm distinguish primates from rodents. *Neuroscience, 157,* 637-643.

[16] May, C. A., Lütjen-Drecoll, E. (2002). Morphology of the murine optic nerve. *Invest Ophthalmol Vis Sci., 43,* 2206-2212.

[17] Schlamp, C. L., Li, Y., Dietz, J. A., Janssen, K. T., Nickells, R. W. (2006). Progressive ganglion cell loss and optic nerve degeneration in DBA/2J mice is variable and asymmetric. *BMC Neurosci., 7,* 66.

[18] Howell, G. R., Libby, R. T., Jakobs, T. C., Smith, R. S., Phalan, F. C., Barter, J. W., et al. (2007) Axons of retinal ganglion cells are insulted in the optic nerve early in DBA/2J glaucoma. *J Cell Biol., 179,* 1523-1537.

[19] Lund, R. D. (1965). Uncrossed visual pathways of hooded and albino rats. *Science, 149,* 1506–1507.

[20] Perry, V. H. (1981). Evidence for an amacrine cell system in the ganglion cell layer of the rat retina. *Neuroscience, 6,* 931–944.

[21] Linden, R., Perry, V. H. (1983). Massive retinotectal projection in rats. *Brain Research, 272,* 145–149.

[22] Sauvé, Y., Girman, S. V., Wang, S., Lawrence, J. M., Lund R. D. (2001). Progressive visual sensitivity loss in the Royal College of

Surgeons rat: Perimetric study in the superior colliculus. *Neuroscience, 103,* 51–63.

[23] Sauvé, Y., Girman, S. V., Wang, S., Keegan, D. J., Lund, R. D. (2002). Preservation of visual responsiveness in the superior colliculus of RCS rats after retinal pigment epithelium cell transplantation. *Neuroscience, 114,* 389–401.

[24] Rodiek, R. W. (1979). Visual pathways. *Annual Reviews of Neuroscience, 2,* 193–225.

[25] Williams, R. W., Strom, R. C., Rice, D. S., Goldwitz, D. (1996). Genetic and environmental control of variation in retinal ganglion cell number in mice. *J Neurosci, 16,* 7193–7205.

[26] Drager, U. C., Olsen, J. F. (1981). Ganglion cell distribution in the retina of the mouse. *Investigative Ophthalmology and Visual Science, 20,* 285–293.

[27] Perry, V. H., Henderson, Z., Linden, R. (1983). Postnatal changes in retinal ganglion cell and optic axon populations in the pigmented rat. *J Comp Neurol., 219,* 356-368.

[28] Jeon, C. J., Strettoi, E., Masland, R. H. (1998). The major cell populations of the mouse retina. *J Neurosci., 18,* 8936-8946.

[29] Schmidt, S. L., Vitral, R. W., Linden, R. (2001). Effects of prenatal ionizing irradiation on the development of the ganglion cell layer of the mouse retina. *Int J Dev Neurosci., 19,* 469-473.

[30] Villegas-Pérez, M. P., Vidal-Sanz, M., Rasminsky, M., Bray, G. M., Aguayo, A. J. (1993). Rapid and protracted phases of retinal ganglion cell loss follow in the optic nerve of adult rats. *J of Neurobiology, 24,* 23-36.

[31] Jakobs, T. C., Libby, R. T., Ben, Y., John, S. W., Masland, R. H. (2005). Retinal ganglion cell degeneration is topological but not cell type specific in DBA/2J mice. *Journal of Cell Biology, 171,* 313–325.

[32] Dreher, B., Sefton, A. J., Ni, S. Y., Nisbett, G. (1985). The morphology, number, distribution and central projections of class I retinal ganglion cells in albino and hooded rats. *Brain Behavior and Evolution, 26*, 10–48.

[33] Perry, V. H., Morris, R. J., Raisman, G. (1984). Is Thy-1 expressed only by ganglion cells and their axons in the retina and optic nerve? *J Neurocytol., 13,* 809-824.

[34] Dabin, I., Barnstable, C. J. (1995). Rat retinal Muller cells express Thy-1 following neuronal cell death. *Glia, 14,* 23-32.

[35] Chidlow, G., Casson, R., Sobrado-Calvo, P., Vidal-Sanz, M., and Osborne, N. N. (2005). Measurement of retinal injury in the rat after optic nerve transection: an RT-PCR study. *Mol Vis., 11,* 387-396.

[36] Huang, W., Fileta, J., Guo, Y., Grosskreutz, C. L. (2006). Downregulation of Thy1 in retinal ganglion cells in experimental glaucoma. *Curr Eye Res., 31,* 265-271.

[37] Schlamp, C. L., Johnson, E. C., Li, Y., Morrison, J. C., Nickells, R. W. (2001). Changes in Thy1 gene expression associated with damaged retinal ganglion cells. *Mol Vis. 7,* 192-201.

[38] Soto, I., Oglesby, E., Buckingham, B. P., Son, J. L., Roberson, E. D., Steele, M. R., et al. (2008). Retinal ganglion cells downregulate gene expression and lose their axons within the optic nerve head in a mouse glaucoma model. *J Neurosci., 28,* 548-561.

[39] Ninkina, N. N., Stevens, G. E., Wood, J. N., Richardson, W. D. (1993) A novel Brn3-like POU transcription factor expressed in subsets of rat sensory and spinal cord neurons. *Nucleic Acids Res 21,* 3175–3182.

[40] Badea, T. C., Williams, J., Smallwood, P., Shi, M., Motajo, O., et al. (2012). Combinatorial expression of Brn3 transcription factors in somatosensory neurons: genetic and morphologic analysis. *J Neurosci., 32,* 995–1007.

[41] Qiu, F., Jiang, H., Xiang, M. (2008). A comprehensive negative regulatory program controlled by Brn3b to ensure ganglion cell specification from multipotential retinal precursors. *J Neurosci., 28,* 3392–3403.

[42] Badea, T. C., Cahill, H., Ecker, J., Hattar, S., Nathans, J. (2009). Distinct roles of transcription factors brn3a and brn3b in controlling the development, morphology, and function of retinal ganglion cells. *Neuron, 61,* 852–864.

[43] Galindo-Romero, C., Avilés-Trigueros, M., Jiménez-López, M. et al. (2011). Axotomy-induced retinal ganglion cell death in adult mice: quantitative and topographic time course analyses. *Exp Eye Res, 92,* 377–387.

[44] Nadal-Nicolás, F. M., Jiménez-López, M., Sobrado-Calvo, P., Nieto-Lopez, L., Canovas-Martínez, I., et al. (2009). Brn3a as a marker of retinal ganglion cells: qualitative and quantitative time course studies in naive and optic nerve-injured retinas. *Invest Ophthalmol Vis Sci., 50,* 3860–3868.

[45] Sánchez-Migallón, M. C., Nadal-Nicolas, F. M., Jiménez-López, M, Sobrado-Calvo, P., Vidal-Sanz, M., et al. (2011). Brain derived neurotrophic factor maintains Brn3a expression in axotomized rat retinal ganglion cells. *Exp Eye Res., 92,* 260–267.

[46] García-Valenzuela, E., Gorczyca, W., Darzynkiewiecz, Z., Sharma, S. C. (1994). Apoptosis in adult retinal ganglion cells after axotomy. *J Neurobiology, 25,* 431-438.

[47] Vidal-Sanz, M., Villegas-Pérez, M. P., Bray, G. M., Aguayo, A. J. (1988). Persistent retrograde labeling of adult rat retinal ganglion cells with the carbocyanine Dye diI. *Exp Neurolog., 102,* 92-101.

[48] Germain, F., Fernández, E., de la Villa, P. (2003). Morphometrical analysis of dendritic arborization in axotomized retinal ganglion cells. *Eur J Neurosci., 18,* 1103–1109.

[49] Germain, F., Calvo, M., de la Villa, P. (2004). Rabbit retinal ganglion cell survival after optic nerve section and its effect on the inner plexiform layer. *Exp Eye Res., 78,* 95–102.

[50] Hilbig, H., Schierwagen, A. (1994). Interlayer neurones in the rat superior colliculus: a tracer study using Dil/Di-ASP. *Neuroreport., 5,* 477-480.

[51] Fischer, D., Pavlidis, M., Thanos, S. (2000). Cataractogenic lens injury prevents traumatic ganglion cell death and promotes axonal regeneration both in vivo and in culture. *Invest Ophthalmol Vis Sci., 41,* 3943–3954.

[52] Cheunsuang, O., Morris, R. (2005). Astrocytes in the arcuate nucleus and median eminence that take up a fluorescent dye from the

circulation express leptin receptors and neuropeptide Y Y1 receptors. *Glia, 52,* 228–233.

[53] Germain, F., Istillarte M., Gómez-Vicente, V., Pérez-Rico, C., de la Villa, P. (2013). Electroretinographical and histological study of mouse retina after optic nerve section: a comparison between wild-type and retinal degeneration 1 mice. *Clin Experiment Ophthalmol., 41,* 593-602.

[54] Mansour-Robaey, S., Clarke, D. B., Wang, Y. C., Bray, G. M., Aguayo, A. J. (1994). Effects of ocular injury and administration of brain-derived neurotrophic factor on survival and regrowth of axotomized retinal ganglion cells. *Proc Natl Acad Sci USA, 91,* 1632-1636.

[55] Sellés-Navarro, I., Villegas-Pérez, M. P., Salvador-Silva, M., Ruiz-Gómez, J. M., Vidal-Sanz, M. (1996). Retinal ganglion cell death after different transient periods of pressure-induced ischemia and survival intervals. A quantitative in vivo study. *Invest Ophthalmol Vis Sci., 37,* 2002-2014.

[56] Vidal-Sanz, M., Lafuente, M. P., Mayor-Torroglosa, S., Aguilera, M. E., Miralles de Imperial, J., Villegas-Pérez, M. P. (2001). Brimonidine's neuroprotective effects against transient ischaemia-induced retinal ganglion cell death. *Eur J Ophthalmol. Suppl. 2,* S36-40.

[57] Lafuente, M. P., Mayor-Torroglosa, S., Miralles de Imperial, J., Villegas-Pérez, M. P., Vidal-Sanz, M. (2002). Transient ischemia of the retina results in altered retrograde axoplamic transport: neuroprotection with brimonidine. *Exp. Neurol., 178*, 243-258.

[58] Paxinos, G., Frankin, K. B. J. (2001). *The Mouse Brain in Stereotaxic Coordinates* 2nd edition. Academic Press, San Diego, California, USA.

[59] Wang, S., Villegas-Pérez, M. P., Vidal-Sanz, M., Lund, R. D. (2000). Progressive optic axon dystrophy and vascular changes in rd mice. *Invest Ophthalmol Vis Sci., 41,* 537–545.

[60] Mabuchi, F., Aihara, M., Mackey, M. R., Lindsey, J. D., Weinreb, R. N. (2004). Regional optic nerve damage in experimental mouse glaucoma. *Invest. Ophthalmol. Vis. Sci., 45,* 4352-4358.

[61] Boycott, B. B., Hopkins, J. M. (1981). Microglia in the retina of monkey and other mammals: its distinction from other types of glia and horizontal cells. *Neuroscience, 6,* 679–688.

[62] Maffei, L., Carmingnoto, G., Perry, V. H., Candeo, P., Ferrari, G. (1990). Schwann cells promote the survival of rat retinal ganglion cells after optic nerve section. *Proc Natl Acad Sci USA, 87,* 1855–1859.

[63] Provis, J. M. (1979). The distribution and size of ganglion cells in the retina of the pigmented rabbit: a quantitative analysis. *J Comp Neurol., 185,* 121–137.

[64] De Juan, J., Iniguez, C., Carreres, J. (1978). Number, diameter and distribution of the rat optic nerve fibers. *Acta Anat (Basel), 102,* 294-299.

[65] Forrester, J., Peters, A. (1967). Nerve fibres in optic nerve of rat. *Nature, 214,* 245-247.

[66] Honjin, R., Sakato, S., Yamashita, T. Electron microscopy of the mouse optic nerve: a quantitative study of the total optic nerve fibers. (1977) *Arch Histol Jpn., 40,* 321-332.

[67] Peinado-Ramón, P., Salvador, M., Villegas-Pérez, M. P., Vidal-Sanz, M. (1996). Effects of axotomy and intraocular administration of NT-4, NT-3, and brain-derived neurotrophic factor on the survival of adult rat retinal ganglion cells. A quantitative in vivo study. *Invest Ophthalmol Vis Sci., 37,* 489-500.

[68] Salinas-Navarro, M., Alarcón-Martínez, L., Valiente-Soriano, F. J., Jiménez-López, M., Mayor-Torroglosa, S., Avilés-Trigueros, M., Villegas-Pérez, M. P., Vidal-Sanz, M. (2010). Ocular hypertension impairs optic nerve axonal transport leading to progressive retinal ganglion cell regeneration. *Exp Eye Res., 90,* 168-83.

[69] Springer, A. D., Wilson, B. R. (1989). Light microscopic study of degenerating cobalt-filled optic axons in goldfish: role of microglia and radial glia in debris removal. *J Comp Neurol., 282,* 119-132.

[70] Cusick, C. G., Lund, R. D. (1982). Modification of visual callosal projections in rats. *J. Comp. Neurol., 212,* 385–398.

[71] Thanos, S. (1991). Specific transcellular carbocyanine-labelling of rat retinal microglia during injury-induced neuronal degeneration. *Neurosci Lett., 127,* 108-112.

[72] Thanos, S., Pavlidis, C., Mey, J., Thiel, H. J. (1992). Specific transcellular staining of microglia in the adult rat after traumatic degeneration of carbocyanine-filled retinal ganglion cells. *Exp Eye Res., 55,* 101-117.

In: Horizons in Neuroscience Research ISBN: 978-1-53613-286-1
Editors: A. Costa and E. Villalba

Chapter 7

A NEUROSCIENCE APPROACH TO SENSITIVE PERIODS IN THE DEVELOPMENT OF A CHILD

Celestyna Grzywniak**, *PhD
Pedagogical University of Cracow, Poland

SENSITIVE PERIODS

ABSTRACT

The aim of the article is to present the basics of neurobiology and neuropsychology, learning processes and forming of neural connections in the brain

The author of the article utilizes knowledge of neurobiology and neuropsychology which are currently part of neuroscience. She describes sensitive periods, also referred to as critical, as periods during which particular neural networks grow more rapidly and numerous synaptic connections are formed. What occurs then is synaptogenesis, which is the base of development of links among cells making the brain more flexible and capable of learning faster. Then she describes the process of learning on the neurophysiological level. The author highlights certain critical

* Corresponding Author: Email: gcel@poczta.onet.pl; Tel: +48 504 384 023.

periods in the development of children. They include touch sensitivity, recognizing faces, sound categorization leading to language learning, ability to count and motion sensitivity. Further in the article, the author refers to the concept of Maria Montessori, which, in certain aspects, is consistent with the occurrence of sensitive periods. Celestyna Grzywniak emphasizes the significance of early teaching of children and enriching their environment by introducing appropriate activities. She draws attention to stimulation of neural links through environment, which should be specially enriched by applying appropriate stimuli. The article emphasizes the need to repeatedly apply effective stimuli in order to enhance the flow of nerve impulses and clear up nerve pathways.

Keywords: neuroscience, sensitive periods, critical periods, neural networks, learning at the neurophysiological level, neural circuits

A Neuroscience Approach to Sensitive Periods

Studies of sensitive periods are the subject-matter of neuroscience. Sensitive periods, also frequently referred to as critical periods, are time brackets, in which certain neural networks grow more rapidly, and also such, during which numerous synaptic connections are formed. In this periods, the process of synaptogenesis is intensified, and the process of learning progresses rapidly and effortlessly. The result is the development of skills and abilities organized by these neural networks and so, new neural networks are formed creating the structure of the brain. During this period, the environment needs to provide appropriate stimuli, which can encourage the child to be active and stimulate the functions of the central nervous system (CNS). Today's science distinguishes several sensitive periods. Those most widely known include: sensitivity to touch, recognizing faces, language learning and many more.

The pioneer of neuroscience studies was Michael S. Gazzaniga, a Nobel Prize laureate. He defined neuroscience as a science studying the manner in which the brain forms the mind (Jaśkowski, P., 2009). It investigates the development of connections between the nerve cells, and also the influence exerted by the environment upon the formation of the brain. A part of neuroscience is constituted by various disciplines concerned with investigations into the brain, such as neurobiology, neuropsychology, neurology or neurophysiology, and others. The neural connections between the cells are referred to as the neural networks, which constitute the neural circuits responsible for learning certain abilities. There are many such circuits in the brain. The neurons in these systems are capable of reorganizing themselves, forming new connections and arborization. Under the influence exerted by learning and stimulation, the neural cell forms new axons in the form of dendrites and numerous synapses by means of which it connects with other cells in the system forming neural networks. Those are composed of trillions of neural connections with various arbors. The individual neural networks may connect with other networks, making it possible for them to undergo integration and to reach a higher level of functioning. The more synaptic arbors and connections, the more efficient and more rapid the transfer of an impulse is, and the stronger the neural pathway is.

These connections are formed thanks to the formation of the synapses in the neural cells. Synaptogenesis, as well as the reduction of the synapses, occurs in the development of the brain throughout the entire life, but, particularly during sensitive periods, in which an intensive development of intersynaptic connections and formation of new neural circuits, frequently referred to as neural networks, occurs. These processes progress most intensively in the period of childhood and early young age. Until reaching the stage of adulthood, the brain will have lost approximately 50% of the redundant and unused synapses. The process of the reduction of the synapses is intensive in the period of young age, thanks to which the circuits which are used more frequently are strengthened and consolidated. This mechanism is the foundation for neural plasticity, making it possible to reorganize the brain. During sensitive periods, environmental stimulation exerts a strong influence upon the formation of the neural networks. The sensual experiences acquired in this period cause permanent and broad-scope changes in the connections of the neural circuits in certain regions of the brain. Environmental stimulation is essential for the growth and the development of the brain.

LEARNING ON NEUROPHYSIOLOGICAL LEVEL

The association areas in the cerebral cortex connect, coordinate and control the multiple neural circuits they are connected to. In order to make sure that the synapses and the axons of a neural cell do not disappear, the stimuli coming from the environment have to be repeated. The frequency of repetitions depends on the kind of the network and other factors, such as the longevity of connections and their strength. In practical terms, one may say that there are adult individuals or children who, having seen, heard or read something once, can retain it in their memory for an extended period of time. In turn, other individuals need multiple repetitions to remember a given utterance. Under the influence exerted by environmental stimulation, the connections in the networks are constantly changing and shaping. Therefore, it is important that the environment is rich in various stimuli, because it builds the appropriate architecture of the brain. Learning is the process of the formation of neural networks, their strengthening and integration, and of the formation of new connections. That process is possible throughout the entire life, but it occurs most rapidly in sensitive periods, and also while the connections between the structures of the brain are forming.

Learning on the neurophysiological level consists of forming of the new synapses and strengthening them by means of the repetition of these processes. Multiple repetitions of these processes make the synapses stronger and more permanent. The longevity of the trace will be dependent upon the number of repetitions, and also upon emotions and motivations. Therefore, a child has to repeat a play a lot of times in order to make the trace in the neural circuits permanent. At the neurophysiological level, in accordance with the opinion of Zofia Kułakowska (Kułakowska, Z., 2003, p. 132) Learning consists of:

- the acquisition of new information by the central nervous system (CNS),
- the formation of internal representations of sensations in the central nervous system

or

- transforming these representations under the influence of experiences.

The process of learning is the capability of making plastic structural and functional changes in the central nervous system, lasting throughout the entire life. In turn, memory involves storing these internal mental representations in time'.

Investigations into the influence exerted by an enriched environment upon the development of the central nervous system indicate that animals living in cages in which they were provided with various levers, swings, balls and obstacle courses, etc., and that means they lived in an environment enriched by various stimuli had a larger number of neurons, synaptic connections, as well as the number of the capillaries, and an increased activity of mitochondria. They were more fidgety, and more willing to engage into playing, and they reacted more rapidly to external stimulation. Animals living in an environment deficient in stimuli, and that means in empty single-colour cages, had a smaller number of synaptic connections and arborizations, and also that their nerve cells, and the neural networks were definitely more deficient, whereas the animals themselves were dejected and reluctant to engage into playing. In the case of human beings, the environment rich in various stimuli provides various opportunities for learning, for the acquisition of new experiences, and also abilities, and broadening their knowledge. The neurons which are frequently stimulated may grow and adapt the neighbouring cells of the nervous system to their tasks. The neural networks develop in the course of learning and facing various challenges from the environment (quoted after: Grzywniak, C., 2017a).

S. J. Blakemore and U. Frith (2008) adhere to the opinion that in sensitive periods the brain is more susceptible to formation and modification under the influence exerted by experiences. In certain periods of life, the brain has to receive appropriate information from the environment, and appropriate stimulation has to occur in the particular stadium of development. These periods are not rigid or inflexible.

Nevertheless, one ought to emphasize that, in these periods, a high level of metabolism occurs, and the circulation of blood through a given structure in the brain is more intensive, and an increase in the consumption of glucose is observed. The time of the occurrence of sensitive periods varies for particular neural systems. Because of that fact, various abilities appear in the course of various periods. Learning during sensitive periods exerts a stronger influence upon the formation of the neural structure, and upon behaviour than experience from the periods which are not sensitive. These periods are genetically-programmed, and they occur when a child reaches a certain age. Various studies show that the formation of the neural networks is influenced, to a considerable extent, by experience and the environment. It is stimuli from the environment that shape the experience of a child, and, *ipso facto*, exert influence upon the formation of the new neural circuits (Szeląg, E., 2015). Learning, and, therefore, the formation of the neural networks is possible throughout the entire life, but it is in the course of childhood that it is rapid and strong, particularly in the pre-verbal period. For that very reason, these neural networks can hardly be modified, and the influence exerted by the experiences from that period leaves a mark lasting throughout the entire life.

Specifying Sensitive Periods in a Child's Development

One of the first sensitive periods which is observed in the case of a child is sensitivity to touch. The sense of touch appears and develops prior to that of eyesight, and the former constitutes the first method of learning, because contact with a neonate occurs in this very manner. By means of touch, we shape the feeling of safety and influence the development of emotions. It is for that reason that it is so important to stroke a child, nurse and hug softly, and also to rock the child. In the early period of development, touching, stroking, turning and rocking are the basis for further correct psychomotor development. By means of rocking, the vestibular system and the connections between it and other systems are developed. The vestibular system is developed quite early, namely as soon as in the sixteenth week of life, and when a child is born, it is prepared for functioning. Infants in the case of whom the vestibular system is systematically stimulated by means of systematic rocking, develop better, and the regular cycle of sleeping is developed earlier, and they also sleep more peacefully. Our grandmothers intuitively arrived at the same conclusion, and it was for that reason that they used cradles when looking after their children. The receptors of the tactile system cover the entire body, and send impulses to the various structures of the nervous system. In this manner, they exert influence upon the formation of various neural connections, and also upon the strengthening of the appropriate neural networks in the entire central nervous system. The feeling of safety and the development of emotions exert influence upon the formation of personality. Childhood deficient in nursing and/or stroking motivated by love may result even in death, or in the formation of psychopathological personality, or another one the structure of which will be incorrect. Emotional development exerts influence upon social development, and is the basis for the correct psychomotor development of a child. The tactile system has to develop early, because upon the basis of this system, the following reflexes: palm-chin, plantar, sucking, looking and Moro are developed.

The subsequent sensitive period is that of differentiating between faces. Until the sixth month of life, an infant recognizes various kinds of faces well, and is capable of telling the difference even between the faces of apes, which is more difficult for adult individuals. Nevertheless, after the sixth month of life, the level of this skill gradually decreases. In turn, at that age children are capable of dealing even better with telling the difference between human faces. The reason for that development is that an infant is principally in contact with human faces. Through observation, it can learn to recognize emotions from facial expressions. Later in life, it can be helpful in developing empathy.

That is compatible with the discovery of the fact that infants are more sensitive to the faces of various species. If an infant stayed among apes or another species, this child would tell the difference between the faces of apes or the animals in the company of whom the child were staying. A similar mechanism applies to speech recognition.

There is also a sensitive period for the categorization of phones, and therefore learning a language. A neonate is capable of telling the difference between the phones of all the languages of the world, and is more sensitive to these phones which makes it possible to tell the difference between one word and another. In this period, children are capable of telling the difference between subtle differences in every language.

Nevertheless, later, the child starts to tell the difference only between these phones which appear in their environment, and which are encountered by the child. At the end of the first year of life, a child loses the skill of telling the difference between these phones which do not occur in their environment; for instance, the Japanese are incapable of telling the difference between the phones: ‘r’ and ‘l’ because those do not occur in their language. Nevertheless, the investigations conducted by Patrycja Kuhl of the University in Seattle in USA in the year 1996 demonstrated that Japanese infants until the tenth month of life are capable of noticing the difference in question. After that period, this skill disappears, because they do not encounter them in their surrounding environment, and lose the ability to tell the difference between them. If Japanese infants living in the USA constantly listened to the Japanese language, this skill would be retained. The investigations demonstrated that the loss of the ability to tell the difference between all phones occurs between 8 and 13 month of life. Prior to this period, infants brought up, for instance, in USA are capable of noticing difference, for instance, between certain sounds of a different language. After this period, this skill disappears. It occurs because in the central nervous system a phonological structure between neural connections forms. Unused synapses disappear. Only those which are strengthened due to being in use remain. When the phonological structure is formed, learning a different language is based upon this ready structure, and, therefore, it is not learning from the scratch any more. For that very reason, the second language is frequently pronounced with a different accent. E. Szeląg (2015) claims that in mid of the second year of life of a child the areas of speech in the left hemisphere enter a sensitive period, and grammatical speech in the left hemisphere is integrating with the interpersonal and prosodic elements of communication, which were earlier developing in the right hemisphere.

When the cortical centres acquire maturity, words join one another, forming sentences. The neurological structure of a language is consolidated, and so is the melody, accent and its rhythm. (quoted after: Grzywniak, C., 2017b).

The subject-matter of the majority of investigations into 'critical periods' concerns the possibility to learn foreign languages by children that emigrated to foreign countries. Investigations into the realm of the correctness of mastering the second language in the case of emigrants demonstrated that it is dependent upon the age at which they commenced learning the second language. It was not different from the pronunciation of the Americans in the case of 68% of individuals that had arrived in USA before the sixth year of their life, in the case of 41% of the individuals that settled there between 7 and 12 year of their lives, and in the case of merely as few as 13% residing there at the age exceeding 19. If the assumption of the occurrence of 'critical periods' is accepted for the development of speech, then it may be presumed that the representation of the language taught at a later age in the brain is different. Other investigations confirmed these presumptions. The investigations were conducted on the Papua people from New Guinea that in various periods of their life emigrated to Australia, and commenced learning the English language there. Investigations into the brain demonstrated that in the course of recognizing words in the English language, the pattern observed is not a homogeneous one. A typical domination of the left hemisphere was observed in the case of these individuals that had settled in Australia before the eighth year of their life, and in the case of individuals that arrived there later, between 9 and 12 year of their life, right-hemisphere specialization occurred. Those results indicate a different mental representations of a foreign language acquired by older children (Szeląg, E., 2015).

As it is demonstrated by investigations, between the 18th and the 36th month of life, the connections in the left hemisphere grow intensively, and the sensitive period for learning new words commences. A child learns a language rapidly and effortlessly.

R. Gelman and R. Gallistel adhere to the opinion that a child has the innate skill to learn about quantities and the rules of grammar (S.-J. Blakemore and Frith, U. 2008, Cozolino, L. 2002). In the same manner in which a child is born with the skill to learn a language, they are born with the skill to learn to count. Scientists claim that the brain of a neonate has to be equipped with some kind of a notion of a number, which is developed in the period of pregnancy. The most recent investigations demonstrate that a neonate several days after being born is capable of recognizing the difference between two and three items. The Frenchman, S. Dehaven, adheres to the opinion that an innate notion of a number, so-called module specialized in the identification of quantities exists, passed on in genes, similarly to the manner in which we inherit the visual or aural systems. This conception also explains why some children find it rather difficult to understand the notion of a number, and why they suffer from dyscalculia. In his opinion, this module does not function correctly in their case. Mathematical skills with which young children are born are restricted to very elementary mathematics. Therefore, a child has to develop the innate predispositions to learning mathematics (Blakemore S. J. and Frith, U., 2008).

The cerebral cortex is developed in a non-linear manner. This process is compatible with the re-organization of the brain caused by the increased multiplication of synapses in the frontal lobes. The period of multiplication is followed by the consolidation of the synapses used by the brain, and trimming the synapses which are not used, similarly to the case of an infant. The best periods for learning occur since the birth until the third year of life and since the 10th until the 15th year of life, because it is in these periods that the radical re-organization of the brain and rapid learning occur.

Nevertheless, one may say that learning occurs at every age because the brain is plastic throughout the entire life. The plasticity of the brain means the skill of adapting to new tasks and to the surrounding environment. If we learn a new ability, a new language, a new activity, the brain has to form new synaptic connections and new dendrites.

Simultaneously with the development of the brain, an increase in the quantity of the neural circuits and growing activity of the cortex occur. Those circuits commence functioning in an ever more synchronized manner. In the early period of life, close relationships with a care-providing individual are also formed, which shape, in the case of a child, the feeling of safety and the matrix of attachment. A period which is particularly sensitive for the formation of these neural networks are the first years of life. In sensitive periods, growth of the neurons and their organization are more intensified, and it is for that reason that early experiences and sensations exert a major influence upon the further life of a child. Those are extra verbal and coeliac sensations, and it increases their resistibility to change. The organized neural networks contain the structures of our early experience, which exerts a much stronger influence upon our life than the further ones do.

In the first two years, the connections between the subcortical centres and cortical centres are developing intensively. In this period, the right hemisphere is developed more rapidly than the left one. In this period, the former one specializes in organizing and receiving experiences from the body, and also in visual-spatial activities, whereas the left one in understanding and expressing speech. By the end of the second year of life, the intensive development of the left hemisphere is commenced, which brings forth the fruit of the intensified development of speech, and mastering the substantial number of words (Cozolino, L., 2002). The right hemisphere also shows more connections with the limbic system and the stem of the brain, which results in the fact that in the case of a substantial stress, impulses from the stem of the brain and from the right hemisphere are blocked, and we are incapable of 'forcing a word to leave out mouth'. Developing differences in the rapidity of the development of both of the hemispheres of the brain is one of the most recent accomplishments of neurophysiology. The development of the right hemispheres at nursery-school age is more rapid than that of the left one. In the right hemisphere, the musical centre and the visual-imaginary centre are situated, and, therefore, a child finds it easier to learn various songs and has a lot of imagination. In this period, music and rhythm support the process of memorizing, which ought to be taken advantage of in the process of learning, for instance, of the multiplication table and of new words.

A child ought to sing a lot, and the multiplication table ought to be sung so as to make it possible for melody to help memorize it. It is less difficult to recall a melody and a rhythm than words not accompanied by either of those two, which mean nothing for a child. It is similarly with the development of a language. As I have already mentioned, the right hemisphere develops slightly earlier in this period. A child memorizes melody and rhythm effortlessly. The melodies of songs for children are accompanied by simpler words. Those words may be divided into syllables in a manner which does not require any efforts. Open syllables dominate.

The rhythm of a song helps to divide words into syllables. By means of dividing the words into syllables, a child practices phonemic hearing, and starts to separate the smallest unit of a word which is a syllable. A child shapes aural analysis and synthesis on the smallest units, and, therefore, on syllables. A child is aided in it by melody and rhythm. Without melody and rhythm, a child at this age is not capable of achieving the skill in question. If a child does not attend nursery school in which a teacher sings with children, dances with them, and also taps the rhythm with legs and clap hands, phonemic hearing may not develop correctly. Singing and dancing provide basis for the development of the language of a child, and, *ipso facto*, for the development of the left hemisphere. In nursery schools, it is nowadays frequent to organize classes of logorythmics, which perfectly develop neural connections between the various centres in the right hemisphere, and in the left one alike (Grzywniak C. 2017).

Additional Development Stages (Sensitive Periods) According to Maria Montessori

As it can be seen, psychomotor development does progress in a harmonious manner, but rather in phases. A similar position in her method was adapted, at the beginning of the twentieth century, by Maria Montessori. She presumed that every child is different, nevertheless, it is possible to notice certain repeating periods in their development frequently referred to as sensitive phases. Those are phases in the course of which it is particularly interested in the selected elements of the environment. Then, the element is subjected to 'processing', and used by children in playing in numerous manners. Children ask many questions then. This interest is not a long-lasting one, and after this time, it starts paying attention to a different item. And in this manner, it acquires more abilities and knowledge about the world surrounding them. All those phases are connected with each other, and concluding one is the starting point for commencing the subsequent one. In the period of the occurrence of certain sensitivity to the acquisition of a given ability, a child experiences a lot of joy due to the activity and unusual enthusiasm in the course of repeating movements or playing. A child demonstrates a strong motivation in the course of the performance of activities, learns easily and effortlessly. If the period of interest in a given activity is concluded, learning this activity in the further period will consume more time and it will require directing one's will in a conscious manner, if that is to be mastered. Maria Montessori by means of observation determined the occurrence of some sensitive phases in the case of children. Those are as follows:

- since 1,5 until the 3rd year of life there occurs the phase of the development of a language
- since 1,5 until the 4th year of life – this is the phase of the development of motor coordination and of the development of muscles
- since the 2nd until the 4th year of life – the phase of perfecting movements
- since the 2nd until the 4th year of life – the phase of ordering and maintaining order
- since 2,5 until the 6th year of life – the phase of perfecting senses
- since the 3rd until the 6th year of life – the phase of susceptibility to the influence exerted by adult individuals

- since the 3,5 until the 4th year of life – the phase of being interested in writing
- since the 4th until 4,5 years of life – willingness to touch items and the development of the sense of touch
- since 4,5 years of life until 5,5 years of life – being interested in reading

Prior to the occurrence of the phase of the development of a language, a child has to undergo the preparatory period in the form of becoming familiar with human speech, the prosody of that, and also preparing articulation organs for speaking in the form of babbling and the previous stage of speech development. After this period, there occurs the assimilation of words. A child in a natural manner, effortlessly and rapidly acquires human speech. The following phase is that of sensitivity to movement. A child has to run, walk and jump in order to learn precise motor activities. Playing is accompanied by grasping items, manipulating and carrying them to a different place, throwing, catching and passing. Motor playing makes a child feel joyful, and practised capacities are perfected at a surprising rapidity. At this age, there also occurs the phase of the development of order. The awareness of order is developed, and so is that of putting items on their proper places, matching them to their appropriate places. The phase of ordering helps to understand reality, provides the feeling of safety and helps acquire harmony, both external and internal one alike. A child begins to understand that items have their appropriate places, and that they ought to be put there. Activities throughout the day have to be performed in accordance with the determined sequence and a non-changeable plan. Montessori considers this phase to be very important, because it helps to order the hitherto acquired experiences and constitutes the basis for collecting further impressions. The phase of perfecting senses is the period of increased sensual sensitivity. Children are willing to engage in playing, in which they utilize various sensual modalities. In this manner, they subject them to training. Simultaneously, they observe adult individuals, follow their examples and imitate their behaviour. Sensitivity and being interested in writing is commenced quite early because at the age of three and a half years, but it lasts for quite a short time. A child is quite willing to write and draw, and starts asking about letters, and attempts to copy their shape in drawings. After that phase, a child starts to be interested in reading. The child does it with passion. In a traditional school, learning to read and write is commenced at the age of 7 years of life. From the point of view of theoretical bases developed by Montessori, that ought to occur earlier, and, therefore at nursery school age (Montessori, M., 2005, Miksza, M., 2007).

THE NEED OF EARLY TEACHING AND ENRICHING THE CHILD'S ENVIRONMENT

In the period until the sixth 6 year of their life, and since the 10th until the 15th year of life, there occurs rapid learning, because of the simultaneous process of the organization of the brain, and also the consolidation of the neural connections. The neural networks constituting the basis for correct learning are formed. Taking advantage of the potential of the brain in sensitive periods for the purpose of the stimulation of the formation of the neural networks would be more important. In accordance with discoveries in the realm of neuroscience, the education of a child ought to be commenced earlier. The following discoveries in the realm of neurobiology support this view:

- there is a growing number of the connections between the nerve cells in the brains of younger children, and it results in a more rapid learning, broader manner of seeing problems which are formulated in the process of learning, and afterwards better functioning in reality
- there are critical periods in the development of the central nervous system
- the environment rich in positive stimuli causes the formation of the larger number of neural connections in the brain.

- enriching the environment with various stimuli stimulates the growth of neurons and their integration, which, results in easier and more rapid learning
- a child learning appropriate ability in a sensitive period does it with joy and passion, and learning progresses rapidly and without a greater effort in that case.

References

Ayres, J., (1986). *Sensory Integration and Learning Disorders.* Los Angeles, Western Psychological Services, California.

Blakemore, S., Frith U., (2008). *How a brain learns.* Wydawnictwo Uniwersytetu Jagiellońskiego, Kraków.

Cozolino, L. J., (2002). *The neuroscience of psychotherapy building and rebuilding the human brain.* Copyright by Louis J. Cozolino, New York.

Grzywniak, C., (2017b). Incorrect auditory processing and the functioning of children and adults. Development, upbringing and therapy. *Advances in Psychology Research,* Volume 131, Editor Alexsandra M. Columbus, Published by Nova Science Publishers, Inc. USA, (eBook), 227- 240

Grzywniak, C., (2017a). *Neuropsychological maturity for school education of children at the age of 6 and 7.* Wydawnictwo Scriptum, Kraków.

Grzywniak, C., (2011). Basics of neurobiology in learning of younger children, *Comitee on Education Annual,* Volume LXIV, 95-106.

Grzywniak, C., (2008). Primitive reflexes and the emergence of learning difficulties in children at school age, in (ed.): M. Bogdanowicz, M. Lipowska, *Family, educational and psychological indicators of development,* Impuls, Kraków.

Grzywniak, C., (2017). Seeking therapy methods for children with learning difficulties, *Acta Neuropsychologica;* 15 (3) s.241-255,

Grzywniak, C., (2015). *Development stimulation of children with learning difficulties – new trends*, Wydawnictwo Naukowe Uniwersytetu Pedagogicznego, Kraków.

Jaśkowski, P., (2009). *Cognitive science – how the brain creates the mind, Vizja Press&It,* Warszawa.

Kędzia, A.., (2001). *Structure and functions of the nervous system, in (ed.): L. Sadowska, Neurokinesiological diagnostics and therapy of children with psychomotor development disorders,* Wydawnictwo AWF, Wrocław.

Konturek, S., (1998). *Human neurophysiology, Wydawnictwo Uniwersytetu Jagiellońskiego,* Kraków.

Kułakowska, Z., (2003). *Early damages to a developing brain,* Folium, Lublin.

Longstaff, A., (2009). *Neurobiology,* PWN, Warszawa.

Maas, V., (2007). *Sensor integration and neuroscience– birth to old age,* Fundacja Innowacja i Wyższa Szkoła Społeczno-Ekonomiczna, Warszawa.

Miksza, M., (2007). *Understanding Montessori - Maria Montessori on bringing up children,* Impuls, Kraków.

Montessori, M., (2005). *Children homes,* Wyd. Akademickie Żak, Warszawa.

Szeląg, E., (20015). *Speech mechanics of the brain,* In (ed.): Grabowska A., Asymetria półkul mózgowych, in (ed.): T. Górska, A. Grabowska, J. Zagrodzka, Mózg a zachowanie, PWN, Warszawa.

In: Horizons in Neuroscience Research ISBN: 978-1-53613-286-1
Editors: A. Costa and E. Villalba

Chapter 8

VESSEL WALL MRI AND INTRACRANIAL ANEURYSMS

P. Bhogal*[*], *C. Uff and H. L. D. Makalanda
Department of Neuroradiology, The Royal London Hospital, Whitechapel Road, London, UK

ABSTRACT

Advanced imaging techniques have allowed intracranial aneurysms to be examined under ever-closer scrutiny. Whilst some of these imaging techniques are still at the research stage others have entered clinical practice. One technique in particular holds much promise and could enter routine use in hospital practice with relative ease. This new technique, that allows assessment of the vessel wall and aneurysm wall offers the potential to assess both ruptured and unruptured aneurysms at the level of the wall and underlying pathology that has hitherto been impossible to do with standard luminal imaging techniques such as angiography. In this review we discuss the current knowledge of vessel wall MRI in the assessment of intracranial aneurysms.

Contrast enhanced vessel wall MRI is a state-of –the-art technique that aims to assess the vessel wall and provide real time in vivo

[*] Corresponding Author: Dr. P. Bhogal, Email: bhogalweb@aol.com, Mobile: 07815 937220.

pathological level imaging. To successfully image the intracranial vessel walls one needs to suppress the intra-arterial signal from the blood – the so-called black blood technique. This is essential in order to attain sufficient image contrast to enable accurate assessment and interpretation of the vessel wall. However, this can be a difficult task given that the angulation of the blood vessels is extremely variable which means sufficient suppression of the blood signal can be challenging. A variety of different methods have been used to obtain black blood imaging and these include the use of motion sensitizing pre-pulses [1, 2] and double inversion recovery techniques [3]. It is also important to suppress the CSF signal surrounding the vessels in order to allow a complete assessment of the arterial wall. However, a problem with CSF signal suppression is the resultant decrease in Signal-to-noise ratio (SNR) derived from the vessel wall itself. The combination of multiple suppression sequences and high resolution imaging can also mean prohibitively long scan times and increasing motion artefacts that cause image degradation [4].

The small size of the intracranial vessels and the need for high spatial resolution with high SNR and acceptable scan times necessitates a reduced scan volume. This has in turn resulted in a focus on the circle of Willis and proximal intracranial vessels. Some investigators have opted for a lower spatial resolution to detect enhancement of the vessels secondary to the increase in contrast to noise ratio caused by contrast uptake [5–7]. This approach may be useful to assess the generalised burden and anatomical distribution of a disease process.

As mentioned earlier high SNR is essential for adequate assessment of the vessel wall. The introduction of 3Tesla machines into routine practice has meant improved SNR is now available and this can be used to either shorten scan times or improve spatial resolution [8, 9]. The availability of 7Tesla MR machines, although generally restricted to research institutions at the current time, will hopefully mean further similar improvements in spatial resolution and scan times can be made.

Wall Imaging in Unruptured Aneurysms

The prevalence of unruptured intracranial aneurysm is approximately 3% [10]. Many of these aneurysms are incidentally found on routine scans performed for indications separate to an underlying vascular disease and in these scenarios the discovery of an aneurysm can lead to a considerable degree of stress and anxiety in patients. Studies have determined that a variety of factors can be used to determine the prognosis of these aneurysms and the overall risk of rupture and hence they have formed the basis of treatment guidelines. These factors include the exact location of the aneurysm, either in the anterior or posterior circulation, its size and morphology in addition to a variety of other factors such as gender, ethnicity and age [11]. In the anterior circulation the ISUIA II investigators recommend a size threshold of 7mm as a maximal diameter starting from which intervention should be considered [12, 13]. However, in just over one third of patients that present with subarachnoid haemorrhage (SAH) the source of the bleed is an aneurysm that measures less than 5mm in maximal diameter [14]. Furthermore, in other studies even smaller aneurysms have been seen to rupture. For example in the study of Ishibashi et al. [15], of 19 patients that had a documented rupture during the follow-up period, 14 aneurysms were 5mm or smaller and of these 6 aneurysms were only 3mm in maximal diameter. Therefore, there is a discrepancy in the data where on the one hand the IUSIA data suggest small aneurysms rupture infrequently however, there is considerable evidence that shows small ruptured aneurysms are commonly encountered in clinical practice. It is clear that our understanding of intracranial aneurysms and the factors that lead to aneurysmal growth and rupture is incomplete and the apparent conflict in the literature must be reconciled.

The formation, growth and rupture of aneurysms has been thought to involve inflammation [16]. Before the introduction of contrast-enhanced vessel wall MRI it was difficult to determine whether the inflammatory process seen in the walls of ruptured aneurysms occurred prior to or after the rupture. In order to determine if inflammation could be seen *in vivo* super-paramagnetic iron oxide particles (Ferumyxotol) have been used as a contrast agent. This contrast agent can demonstrate inflammatory activity and using this technique some investigators have shown that inflammation does occur within the walls of some aneurysms. Furthermore, they have shown that circumferential wall uptake in the aneurysm on scans obtained 24-72hours post contrast infusion was highly predictive of aneurysm rupture within the next 6 months [17]. In the study of Hasan et al. of the 6 aneurysms that were being actively watched there were 3 ruptures and each of these aneurysms demonstrated early wall enhancement and were large (15mm in diameter or larger).

The use of vessel wall imaging represents a potential major advance in the ability to analyse intracranial aneurysms. Although size, morphology, anatomical location and a variety of other factors are known to be involved in the prognosis of aneurysms none of these measures assesses the true site of pathology, namely the vessel wall itself. With this in mind Edjlali et al. [18] used this technique to evaluate stable and unstable aneurysms. Unstable aneurysms were defined as those that were symptomatic or evolving in comparison to previous imaging e.g., showed increase in size, new lobulations etc. None of the aneurysms were ruptured at the time of recruitment into the study. In these unstable aneurysms circumferential aneurysmal wall enhancement (CAWE) was seen in 79% of cases (n = 14) whereas CAWE was seen in only 28.5% of patients with stable aneurysms (22/77). This finding was highly statistically significant ($p < 0.0001$). In the study of Nagahata et al. [19] some enhancement was seen in 18% of patients (5% showed strong enhancement and 13% showed faint enhancement). Of the 4 unruptured aneurysms that showed strong enhancement, 2 were unstable with one rapidly increasing in size and the other causing acute third nerve palsy. One of the other aneurysms that showed strong enhancement was 3mm in diameter, indicating both that size alone is not a good indicator of rupture risk and that the technique itself can be used in the assessment of small aneurysms. Hu et al. [20] in their recent publication showed that of the 14 unruptured aneurysms in their cohort, 12 that demonstrated wall enhancement were symptomatic with a strong correlation between aneurysm wall enhancement and symptomatic status on contingency table tests.

In a further recent study Coutinho et al. [21] looked at vessel wall enhancement in patients with angiogram negative non-perimesencephalic subarachnoid haemorrhage. They found that 4 patients showed vessel wall enhancement near potential sites of intracranial arterial rupture that could have been missed on standard luminal imaging. This raises the potential that, in certain scenarios, there are completely obliterated or thrombosed aneurysms that will not be easily detected with standard luminal imaging modalities. Although angiographic imaging is indicated in all cases of SAH, because of the high predictive value of the haemorrhage pattern and CT angiography in peri-mesencephalic haemorrhage (PMH) some authors believe that only a single catheter angiogram is warranted in these patients [22, 23]. However, in cases of non-PMH where a culprit aneurysm is not seen a second catheter angiogram is always indicated since structural abnormalities can be obscured on the initial angiogram and this can occur in between 4-30% of cases [24–27]. Similarly, repeat haemorrhage has been shown to occur in this group of patients [26] therefore, it is important to develop methods to identify early those patients that may be harbouring an occult lesion. A non-invasive imaging modality that would allow both assessment of the vessel lumen and the vessel could act as an excellent screening tool in this cohort of patients.

Vessel Wall MRI in Ruptured Aneurysms

Up to 30% of patients can have more than one aneurysm [28] and in the case of acute rupture this can sometimes pose a diagnostic and treatment dilemma since it is not always clear which aneurysm has ruptured. Various different imaging characteristics have been shown to be associated with a ruptured aneurysm in cases of multiple aneurysms. For example, in a Japanese study of >5000 patients, size, location and presence of a daughter sac were all associated with rupture [29]. Similarly in a Dutch study aneurysm size, aspect ratio, and shape were associated with rupture [30]. A recent Finnish study showed similar findings with both size and irregularity being independently associated with rupture on multivariate analysis and irregularity showing the strongest association with an OR of 90.3 (95% confidence interval 47.0-173.5) [31]. Whilst this information is no doubt useful and certainly assists in targeting the likely ruptured aneurysm errors can still be made especially if the aneurysms are similar in appearance. In the setting of multiple aneurysms and acute SAH the aim is to exclude the ruptured aneurysm from the circulation initially and treat the remaining aneurysms at a later stage. Naturally this can involve endovascular coiling, microsurgical clipping or a combination of both as well as alternative treatment strategies such as parent vessel occlusion. Additionally, there are further issues around which type of procedure should be performed first [32]. Logically the answer to this question revolves around identifying the culprit aneurysm and optimising treatment of this aneurysm first with treatment of the remaining unruptured aneurysms based around best evidence, the local expertise and the patient's wishes.

Irrespective of whether endovascular or microsurgical treatment is used, the optimum strategy would be to treat the aneurysm that has bled and perform delayed treatment on the remaining aneurysms. Vessel wall MRI has been used in this circumstance to guide treatment and Matouk et al. [33] were the first to publish the use of this technique with regards to multiple aneurysms. Of the 5 patients they presented 3 had multiple aneurysms and enhancement was seen in only the ruptured aneurysms. An important point to consider when interpreting this paper is that all the aneurysms were treated endovascularly and although no pathological correlation was obtained there were no repeat haemorrhages, thus it is likely that the culprit aneurysm was successfully treated. This lack of pathological correlation has been overcome in other studies. In the series of Nagahata et al. [19] 15 patients were seen to have enhancement at the apex or on a bleb of the aneurysm. Seven of these 15 cases underwent surgical clipping and in all cases the rupture point correlated with the point of enhancement. Kondo et al. [34] published a further case with two aneurysms associated with evenly distributed subarachnoid blood. In this case the aneurysms arose from the basilar tip and the anterior communicating artery. The basilar tip aneurysm measured 6mm and was the larger of the two, therefore it was believed to be the most likely source of haemorrhage. Vessel wall MR imaging was performed and this revealed thick wall enhancement of the aneurysm arising from the anterior communicating artery and at microsurgical clipping the anterior communicating artery aneurysm was seen to have ruptured. Similarly Hu et al. [20] recently reported their results of 25 patients with 30 aneurysms. They showed that 12/14 symptomatic aneurysms demonstrated wall enhancement and all 6 ruptured aneurysms showed enhancement with 5/6 ruptured aneurysms being <7mm and 2 aneurysms <5mm.

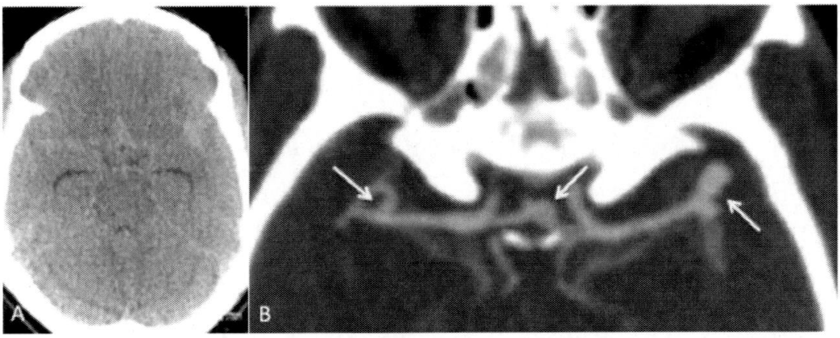

Figure 1. An unenhanced axial CT scan shows widespread subarachnoid haemorrhage (Figure 1a). A CT angiogram was performed which demonstrated 3 aneurysms (Figure 1b, white arrows) the largest being the left MCA bifurcation aneurysm. The culprit aneurysm could not be accurately identified and therefore vessel wall MRI was performed.

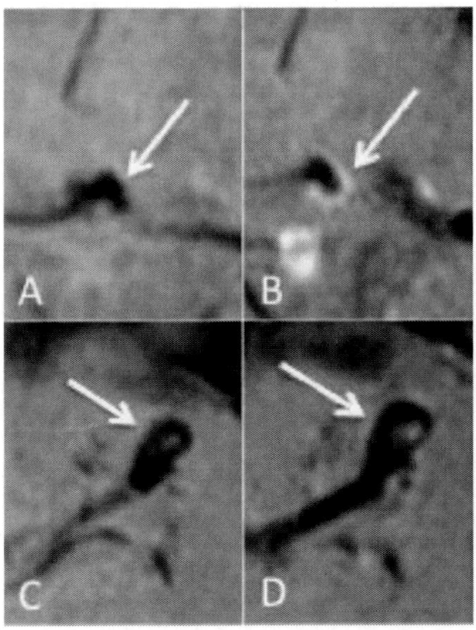

Figure 2. Magnified images of the Acom aneurysms (Figure 2a and 2b) and left MCA (Figure 2c and 2d) pre and post contrast. The avid contrast enhancement of the ACom aneurysm can be clearly seen (Figure 2b) whereas there is no significant enhancement of the left MCA bifurcation aneurysm (Figure 2d).

A similar case was recently seen in our institution [35]. In this case bilateral middle cerebral artery (MCA) bifurcation aneurysms and an aneurysm arising from the anterior communicating (ACom) artery were seen in a patient with acute subarachnoid haemorrhage (Figure 1). The distribution of blood was symmetrical and therefore not helpful in localising the culprit aneurysm. Vessel wall MRI was performed and this showed thick enhancement of the small ACom artery aneurysm and not of the much larger left MCA bifurcation aneurysm (Figure 2). This patient underwent microsurgical clipping and the ACom artery aneurysm was found to have ruptured (Figure 3).

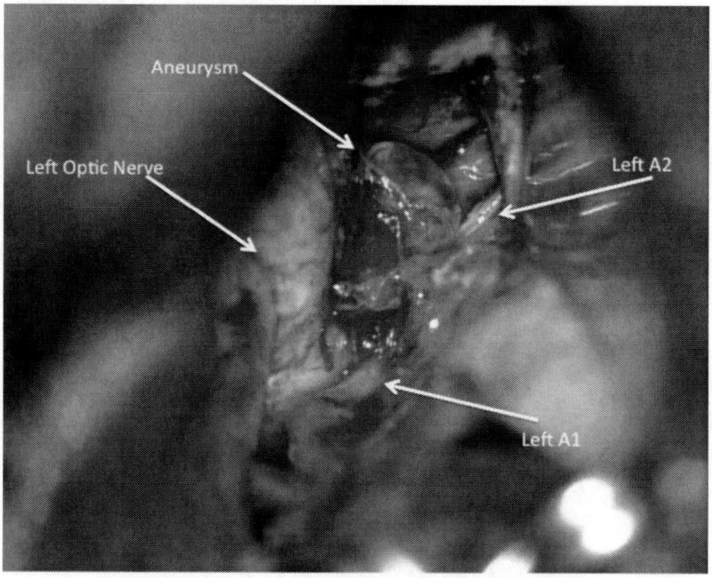

Figure 3. Intraoperative photograph (obtained from Zeiss Pantero 900 surgical microscope). Adjacent to the ACom aneurysm haemorrhagic brain was seen and during deployment of the clip the aneurysm ruptured again. This was controlled with full clip deployment.

Large long-term studies are yet to be performed however, the current studies suggest a high sensitivity and specificity for the detection of aneurysmal rupture. The study by Nagahata et al. [19] gave a sensitivity of 98.4% and specificity of 81.9% with the study of Edjalali et al. [4] gave a sensitivity of 87% and specificity of 71.4%.

CONCLUSION

Technological advancements provide diagnostic and interventional neuroradiologists with more tools to accurately diagnose and manage patients with aneurysms and subarachnoid haemorrhage. The use of vessel wall MR imaging allows us to start analysing aneurysms at a pathophysiological level and not just at an anatomical level. The technology required to perform vessel wall MR imaging is within reach of most hospitals with dedicated neurosurgical and neuro-interventional services. We believe that the advent and acceptance of this technology will assist clinicians and interventional neuroradiologists and allow them to make more personalised treatment decisions based on pathophysiological processes rather than anatomical features alone.

CONFLICT OF INTEREST

There are no conflicts of interest to declare.

DATA SHARING

There is no further data or information available to share at this time.

FUNDING

This research received no specific grant from any funding agency in the public, commercial or not-for-profit sectors.

REFERENCES

[1] Koktzoglou I, Kirpalani A, Carroll TJ, et al. Dark-blood MRI of the thoracic aorta with 3D diffusion-prepared steady-state free precession: initial clinical evaluation. *AJR Am J Roentgenol* 2007;189:966–72. doi:10.2214/AJR.07.2428.

[2] Wang J, Yarnykh VL, Hatsukami T, et al. Improved suppression of plaque-mimicking artifacts in black-blood carotid atherosclerosis imaging using a multislice motion-sensitized driven-equilibrium (MSDE) turbo spin-echo (TSE) sequence. *Magn Reson Med Off J Soc Magn Reson Med Soc Magn Reson Med* 2007;58:973–81. doi:10.1002/mrm.21385.

[3] Swartz RH, Bhuta SS, Farb RI, et al. Intracranial arterial wall imaging using high-resolution 3-tesla contrast-enhanced MRI. *Neurology* 2009;72:627–34. doi:10.1212/01.wnl.0000342470.69739.b3.

[4] Edjlali M, Gentric J-C, Régent-Rodriguez C, et al. Does Aneurysmal Wall Enhancement on Vessel Wall-MRI Help to Distinguish Stable From Unstable Intracranial Aneurysms? *Stroke* 2014; STROKEAHA.114.006626. doi:10.1161/STROKEAHA.114.006626.

[5] Klein IF, Lavallée PC, Schouman-Claeys E, et al. High-resolution MRI identifies basilar artery plaques in paramedian pontine infarct. *Neurology* 2005;64:551–2. doi:10.1212/01.WNL.0000150543.61244.06.

[6] Li M, Xu W, Song L, et al. Atherosclerosis of middle cerebral artery: evaluation with high-resolution MR imaging at 3T. *Atherosclerosis* 2009;204:447–52. doi:10.1016/j.atherosclerosis.2008.10.019.

[7] Turan TN, Bonilha L, Morgan PS, et al. Intraplaque hemorrhage in symptomatic intracranial atherosclerotic disease. *J Neuroimaging Off J Am Soc Neuroimaging* 2011;21:e159-161. doi:10.1111/j.1552-6569.2009.00442.x.

[8] Qiao Y, Steinman DA, Qin Q, et al. Intracranial arterial wall imaging using three-dimensional high isotropic resolution black blood MRI at

3.0 Tesla. *J Magn Reson Imaging JMRI* 2011;34:22–30. doi:10.1002/jmri.22592.

[9] Qiao Y, Etesami M, Astor BC, et al. Carotid plaque neovascularization and hemorrhage detected by MR imaging are associated with recent cerebrovascular ischemic events. *AJNR Am J Neuroradiol* 2012;33:755–60. doi:10.3174/ajnr.A2863.

[10] Vlak MH, Algra A, Brandenburg R, et al. Prevalence of unruptured intracranial aneurysms, with emphasis on sex, age, comorbidity, country, and time period: a systematic review and meta-analysis. *Lancet Neurol* 2011;10:626–36. doi:10.1016/S1474-4422(11)70109-0.

[11] Wermer MJH, Schaaf IC van der, Algra A, et al. Risk of Rupture of Unruptured Intracranial Aneurysms in Relation to Patient and Aneurysm Characteristics An Updated Meta-Analysis. *Stroke* 2007;38:1404–10. doi:10.1161/01.STR.0000260955.51401.cd.

[12] Wiebers DO, Whisnant JP, Huston J, *et al.* Unruptured intracranial aneurysms: natural history, clinical outcome, and risks of surgical and endovascular treatment. *Lancet Lond Engl* 2003;362:103–10.

[13] Unruptured intracranial aneurysms--risk of rupture and risks of surgical intervention. International Study of Unruptured Intracranial Aneurysms Investigators. *N Engl J Med* 1998;339:1725–33. doi:10.1056/NEJM199812103392401.

[14] Juvela S, Porras M, Poussa K. Natural history of unruptured intracranial aneurysms: probability of and risk factors for aneurysm rupture. *J Neurosurg* 2000;93:379–87. doi:10.3171/jns.2000.93.3.0379.

[15] Ishibashi T, Murayama Y, Urashima M, et al. Unruptured intracranial aneurysms: incidence of rupture and risk factors. *Stroke J Cereb Circ* 2009;40:313–6. doi:10.1161/STROKEAHA.108.521674.

[16] Chalouhi N, Hoh BL, Hasan D. Review of cerebral aneurysm formation, growth, and rupture. *Stroke J Cereb Circ* 2013;44:3613–22. doi:10.1161/STROKEAHA.113.002390.

[17] Hasan D, Chalouhi N, Jabbour P, et al. Early Change in Ferumoxytol-Enhanced Magnetic Resonance Imaging Signal

Suggests Unstable Human Cerebral Aneurysm. A Pilot Study. *Stroke J Cereb Circ* 2012;43:3258–65. doi:10.1161/STROKEAHA.112.673400.

[18] Edjlali M, Gentric J-C, Régent-Rodriguez C, et al. Does aneurysmal wall enhancement on vessel wall MRI help to distinguish stable from unstable intracranial aneurysms? *Stroke J Cereb Circ* 2014;45:3704–6. doi:10.1161/STROKEAHA.114.006626.

[19] Nagahata S, Nagahata M, Obara M, et al. Wall Enhancement of the Intracranial Aneurysms Revealed by Magnetic Resonance Vessel Wall Imaging Using Three-Dimensional Turbo Spin-Echo Sequence with Motion-Sensitized Driven-Equilibrium: A Sign of Ruptured Aneurysm? *Clin Neuroradiol* Published Online First: 21 October 2014. doi:10.1007/s00062-014-0353-z.

[20] Hu P, Yang Q, Wang D-D, et al. Wall enhancement on high-resolution magnetic resonance imaging may predict an unsteady state of an intracranial saccular aneurysm. *Neuroradiology* 2016;58:979–85. doi:10.1007/s00234-016-1729-3.

[21] Coutinho JM, Sacho RH, Schaafsma JD, et al. High-Resolution Vessel Wall Magnetic Resonance Imaging in Angiogram-Negative Non-Perimesencephalic Subarachnoid Hemorrhage. *Clin Neuroradiol* Published Online First: 25 November 2015. doi:10.1007/s00062-015-0484-x.

[22] Kaim A, Proske M, Kirsch E, et al. Value of repeat-angiography in cases of unexplained subarachnoid hemorrhage (SAH). *Acta Neurol Scand* 1996;93:366–73.

[23] Rinkel GJ, van Gijn J, Wijdicks EF. Subarachnoid hemorrhage without detectable aneurysm. A review of the causes. *Stroke* 1993;24:1403–9.

[24] Juul R, Fredriksen TA, Ringkjøb R. Prognosis in subarachnoid hemorrhage of unknown etiology. *J Neurosurg* 1986;64:359–62. doi:10.3171/jns.1986.64.3.0359.

[25] Pathirana N, Refsum SE, McKinstry CS, et al. The value of repeat cerebral angiography in subarachnoid haemorrhage. *Br J Neurosurg* 1994;8:141–6.

[26] Nishioka H, Torner JC, Graf CJ, et al. Cooperative study of intracranial aneurysms and subarachnoid hemorrhage: a long-term prognostic study. III. Subarachnoid hemorrhage of undetermined etiology. *Arch Neurol* 1984; 41:1147–51.

[27] Iwanaga H, Wakai S, Ochiai C, et al. Ruptured cerebral aneurysms missed by initial angiographic study. *Neurosurgery* 1990; 27:45–51.

[28] Juvela S. Risk factors for multiple intracranial aneurysms. *Stroke J Cereb Circ* 2000; 31:392–7.

[29] UCAS Japan Investigators, Morita A, Kirino T, et al. The natural course of unruptured cerebral aneurysms in a Japanese cohort. *N Engl J Med* 2012; 366:2474–82. doi:10.1056/NEJMoa1113260.

[30] Backes D, Vergouwen MDI, Velthuis BK, et al. Difference in aneurysm characteristics between ruptured and unruptured aneurysms in patients with multiple intracranial aneurysms. *Stroke J Cereb Circ* 2014; 45:1299–303. doi:10.1161/STROKEAHA.113.004421.

[31] Björkman J, Frösen J, Tähtinen O, et al. Irregular Shape Identifies Ruptured Intracranial Aneurysm in Subarachnoid Hemorrhage Patients With Multiple Aneurysms. *Stroke* Published Online First: 3 May 2017. doi:10.1161/STROKEAHA.117.017147.

[32] Choudhri O, Mukerji N, Steinberg GK. Combined endovascular and microsurgical management of complex cerebral aneurysms. *Front Neurol* 2013; 4:108. doi:10.3389/fneur.2013.00108.

[33] Matouk CC, Mandell DM, Günel M, et al. Vessel wall magnetic resonance imaging identifies the site of rupture in patients with multiple intracranial aneurysms: proof of principle. *Neurosurgery* 2013; 72:492–496; discussion 496. doi:10.1227/NEU.0b013e31827d1012.

[34] Kondo R, Yamaki T, Mouri W, et al. [Magnetic resonance vessel wall imaging reveals rupture site in subarachnoid hemorrhage with multiple cerebral aneurysms]. *No Shinkei Geka* 2014; 42:1147–50. doi:10.11477/mf.1436200050.

[35] Bhogal P, Uff C, Makalanda HLD. Vessel wall MRI and intracranial aneurysms. *J Neurointerventional Surg* Published Online First: 19 November 2015. doi:10.1136/neurintsurg-2015-012130.

In: Horizons in Neuroscience Research
Editors: A. Costa and E. Villalba
ISBN: 978-1-53613-286-1

Chapter 9

CEREBRAL ANEURYSM REBLEEDING

Stephanie H. Chen, MD, Omar S. Elwardany MSc, Samir Sur, MD and Robert M. Starke*, MD

Department of Neurological Surgery & Radiology,
University of Miami, Miami, FL, US

ABSTRACT

Aneurysmal rebleeding after initial subarachnoid hemorrhage is associated with very high morbidity and mortality. While some studies suggest rebleeding occurs in approximately 4% of patients within the first 24 hours after initial subarachnoid hemorrhage, these studies may have underestimated the incidence of ultra-early rebleeding. Furthermore, there remains significant controversy regarding the risk factors, pathophysiology and optimal treatment to prevent rebleeding. In this chapter we summarize the current knowledge on the timing, risk factors and management of aneurysmal rebleeding.

* Corresponding Author: Robert Starke, MD, MSc, Department of Neurological Surgery & Radiology, Miami University, Lois Pope LIFE Center, 1095 N.W. 14th Terrace, 2nd Floor, (D4-6), Miami, FL 33136-1060, Tel: (305) 355-1102, Fax: (305) 355-1102, RStarke@med.miami.edu.

Keywords: cerebral aneurysm, rebleeding, aneurysm rerupture, ultra-early rebleeding, antifibrinolytic therapy, subarachnoid hemorrhage

INTRODUCTION

Although our understanding of cerebral aneurysms and management after rupture has improved dramatically over the years, aneurysmal rebleeding remains an area of considerable interest, and optimal strategy for prevention remains controversial. Repeat aneurysm rupture after initial aneurysmal subarachnoid hemorrhage (SAH) is associated with very high mortality and poor prognosis for functional recovery [1, 2]. Mortality associated with rebleeding has been reported as high as 80% compared to 40% in acute subarachnoid hemorrhage (aSAH) patients [3-6]. Improving our understanding of this phenomenon has the potential to enable better management of these patients and improve the morbidity and mortality associated aneurysmal SAH [7].

INCIDENCE AND TIMING

Aneurysms presenting with subarachnoid hemorrhage are considered high risk due to their tendency to rebleed. The highest risk of rerupture is within the first 2 to 24 hours of symptoms, with rates of occurrence between 4% and 13.6% [3, 4, 8-12]. The risk of rebleeding rises to approximately 15 to 20% within the first two weeks and 30 to 50% for the first 3 months [8-13]. Some studies suggest the majority of rebleeding appears to occur even within the first 6 hours. Tanno et al. reported 48.6% of rebleeding occurred within 6 hours of initial SAH, whereas Okhuma et al. and Cha et al. found a majority of rebleeding occurred within 2 hours of onset, 77% and 74.3% respectively [4-6]. These studies may even underestimate the incidence of ultra-early rebleeding when considering delays from ictus to initial imaging as well as prehospital deaths. Additionally, rebleeding prior to initial CT scan is likely under-reported.

RISK FACTORS AND PREDICTORS

Risk factors associated with aneurysm rebleeding include longer time to treatment, poor Hunt Hess grade on admission, presence of sentinel headaches (severe headaches lasting > 1 hour that did not lead to diagnosis of aSAH), presence of intracerebral or intraventricular hematomas, larger aneurysm size, multiple aneurysms, hyperglycemia systolic blood pressure greater than 160 mmHg and platelet function [3, 4, 10, 11, 12, 14, 15].

Beck et al. suggest that the patients with larger aneurysms and multiple aneurysms likely have more fragile vessel walls that are prone to forming aneurysms as well as rebleeding after rupture. These authors also found that patients with a history of sentinel headache had a 10 fold odds for early rebleeding [14]. However, this relationship necessitates further investigation.

Transmural pressure is the difference between intra-aneurysmal pressure and CSF pressure. Increases in systolic blood pressure may increase transmural pressure beyond the compliance of the hemostatic clot resulting in rebleeding. Thus, there is a general agreement that acute hypertension should be controlled after aSAH, however the blood pressure parameters have not been clearly defined [15]. One meta analysis revealed that systolic blood pressure > 160 mmHg is more closely associated with rebleeding (OR 2.39 95% CI = 1.49–3.84) than a systolic blood pressure >140 mmHg (OR = 1. 44, 95% CI = 0.76–2.73) [16].

Conversely insertion of an external ventricular drain and CSF drainage could result in decreased CSF pressure and thus increase transmural pressure. Although outcomes are have been mixed, there is no clear evidence suggesting increased risk of bleeding with CSF drainage [17-20].

Other factors that are independently associated with aneurysmal subarachnoid hemorrhages that do not seem to affect rebleeding include age, sex, smoking, and location of aneurysm (anterior versus posterior circulation) [3, 4, 11, 12, 14]. Furthermore while development of aneurysms and subsequent SAH are associated with genetic factors, no genetic polymorphism has yet been identified to be associated with rebleeding after aSAH [15]. Little data also exists regarding aneurysm morphological characteristics and re-rupture. However, aneurysm wall irregularity, lobulations, daughter sacs, and aspect ratios have been associated with higher rupture risk and may likely apply to re-rupture as well [21-24].

Many studies over the last three decades have also addressed coagulation and fibrinolysis after SAH [3, 25-28]. After SAH, the site of aneurysm rupture is plugged by a fibrin clot. Studies suggest that rebleeding may be associated with reduced clot stability due to the equilibrium between coagulation cascades and fibrinolysis in the aneurysmal microenvironment [3, 25-28].

The initial event in the coagulation cascade is the release of tissue factor from injured vessel endothelium that causes a thrombin burst. The production of thrombin results in fibrin polymerization and platelet aggregation in the damaged vessels, effectively plugging the site of hemorrhage. A number of studies have examined serum levels of clot modulators in relation to rebleeding [26, 30-33]. Pliego and Muchnik found reduced FXIII activity as well as increased FDP in patients with rebleeding suggesting that patients who rebleed have increased fibrinolysis compared to those who do not [26].

Alternatively, Fujii et al. proposed the “unstable platelet plug hypothesis” wherein rebleeding is associated with decreased platelet aggregability. In their series, using a platelet sensitivity assay they found platelet aggregability level was the strongest independent predictor of ultra-early rebleeding [3]. Juvela and Kaste similarly found decreased thromboxane release, a prostacyclin hormone that induces platelet aggregation and vasoconstriction, in patients with rebleeding after SAH [29].

MEDICAL MANAGEMENT TO PREVENT REBLEEDING AFTER ASAH

Acute hypertension after aSAH should be controlled until aneurysm obliteration, however the optimal parameters for blood pressure control have not been identified. Retrospective data suggests that systolic blood pressure greater than 160 mm Hg might be associated with increased risk of rebleeding, and thus this cutoff point is often used to initialize therapy [4]. Nicardipine and labetolol should be used in conjunction with an arterial line. Hypotension should be avoided to prevent ischemia [15].

Antifibrinolytic therapy has been shown to reduce the rate of rebleeding after aSAH. However, it has also been associated with a marked increase in delayed cerebral ischemia, resulting in no significant difference in functional outcome between those who did and did not receive antifibrinolytic therapy [37-40]. (ISAT) A Cochrane Review in 2013 analyzed ten trials involving 1904 participants. The duration of antifibrinolytic treatment varied considerably between studies ranging form less than 72 hours up to six weeks. Antifibrinolytic therapy significantly reduced the risk of rebleeding (RR 0.65, 95% CI 0.44 to 0.97; 78 per 1000 people), however also significantly increased cerebral ischemia rates (RR 1.41, 95% CI 1.04 to 1.91; 83 per 1000 people). There was no evidence of benefit from antifibrinolytic treatment on case fatality or poor overall outcome [47]. Of note, only one randomized control study by Hillman et al. administered short-term treatment of antifibrinolytics up to 72 hours from presentation, with majority of aneurysms occluded by clipping or coiling within 48 hours of presentation. In this study, rebleeding was significantly reduced in the antifibrinolytics as well as permanent delayed neurologic deficit, suggesting that short-term therapy may lead to improved clinical outcomes [9]. However, further support from large multicenter trials is needed to identify the significance of ultra early antifibrinolytic treatment in overall management. The current American Stroke Association guidelines state, "For patients with an unavoidable delay in obliteration of aneurysm, a significant risk of rebleeding, and no compelling medical contraindications, short-term (< 72 hours) therapy with tranexamic acid or aminocaproic acid is reasonable to reduce the risk of early aneurysm rebleeding [15]." An ongoing prospective randomized control study, The Ultra- Early Tranexamic Acid After Subarachnoid Hemorrhage [ULTRA] trial (NCT02684812), is currently enrolling patients in an effort to answer this question.

SURGICAL AND ENDOVASCULAR MANAGEMENT TO PREVENT REBLEEDING AFTER ASAH

Surgical clipping or endovascular clipping of a ruptured aneurysm should be performed as early as feasible in order to reduce the rate of rebleeding after SAH [15]. While treatment with microsurgical technique versus endovascular approaches remains controversial and unique to the patient population and aneurysm characteristics, in the only multicenter randomized trial comparing microsurgical and endovascular repair, International subarachnoid aneurysm trial, there was no significant difference in early rebleeding rates although overall rebleeding was less common with microsurgical clipping [48].

REFERENCES

[1] Suarez, J. I., Tarr, R. W., Selman, W. R. Aneurysmal subarachnoid hemorrhage. *N. Engl. J. Med.* 2006;354(4):387-96.

[2] Broderick, J. P., Brott, T. G., Duldner, J. E., Tomsick, T., Leach, A. Initial and recurrent bleeding are the major causes of death following subarachnoid hemorrhage. *Stroke.* 1994;25(7):1342-7.

[3] Fujii, Y., Takeuchi, S., Sasaki, O., Minakawa, T., Koike, T., Tanaka, R. Ultra-early rebleeding in spontaneous subarachnoid hemorrhage. *J. Neurosurg.* 1996;84(1):35-42.

[4] Ohkuma, H., Tsurutani, H., Suzuki, S. Incidence and significance of early aneurysmal rebleeding before neurosurgical or neurological management. *Stroke.* 2001;32(5):1176-80.

[5] Cha, K. C., Kim, J. H., Kang, H. I., Moon, B. G., Lee, S. J., Kim, J. S. Aneurysmal rebleeding : factors associated with clinical outcome in the rebleeding patients. *J. Korean Neurosurg. Soc.* 2010;47(2):119-23.

[6] Tanno, Y., Homma, M., Oinuma, M., Kodama, N., Ymamoto, T. Rebleeding from ruptured intracranial aneurysms in North Eastern Province of Japan. A cooperative study. *J. Neurol. Sci.* 2007;258(1-2):11-6.

[7] Rosenorn, J., Eskesen, V., Schmidt, K., Ronde, F. The risk of rebleeding from ruptured intracranial aneurysms. *J. Neurosurg.* 1987;67(3):329-32.

[8] A. Gruber, W. Dietrich, T. Czech, B. Richling. Recurrent aneurysmal subarachnoid haemorrhage: bleeding pattern and incidence of posthaemorrhagic ischaemic infarction. *Br. J. Neurosurg.,* 11 (1997), pp. 121–126.

[9] Hillman, J., Fridriksson, S., Nilsson, O., Yu, Z., Saveland, H., Jakobsson, K. E. Immediate administration of tranexamic acid and reduced incidence of early rebleeding after aneurysmal subarachnoid hemorrhage. *J Neurosurg.* 2002 Oct;97(4):771-8.

[10] T. Inagawa, K. Kamiya, H. Ogasawara, T. Yano Rebleeding of ruptured intracranial aneurysms in the acute stage. *Surg. Neurol.*, 28 (1987), pp. 93–99.

[11] Kitsuta, Y., Suzuki, N., Sugiyama, M., Yamamoto, I. Changes in level of consciousness and association with hyperglycemia as tool for predicting and preventing re-bleeding after spontaneous subarachnoid hemorrhage. *Prehosp. Disaster. Med.* 2006;21(3):190-5.

[12] Naidech, A. M., Janjua, N., Kreiter, K. T., Ostapkovich, N. D., Fitzsimmons, B. F., Parra, A., et al. Predictors and impact of aneurysm rebleeding after subarachnoid hemorrhage. *Arch, Neurol.* 2005;62(3):410-6.

[13] Kassell, N. F., Torner, J. C. Aneurysmal rebleeding: a preliminary report from the Cooperative Aneurysm Study. *Neurosurgery.* 1983 13(5):479-81.

[14] J. Beck, A. Raabe, A. Szelenyi, J. Berkefeld, R. Gerlach, M. Setzer, V. Seifert. Sentinel headache and the risk of rebleeding after aneurysmal subarachnoid hemorrhage. *Stroke,* 37 (2006), pp. 2733–2737.

[15] Connolly, E. S., Jr., Rabinstein, A. A., Carhuapoma, J. R., Derdeyn, C. P., Dion, J., Higashida, R. T., et al. Guidelines for the management of aneurysmal subarachnoid hemorrhage: a guideline for healthcare professionals from the American Heart Association/american Stroke Association. *Stroke.* 2012;43(6):1711-37.

[16] Tang, C., Zhang, T. S., Zhou, L. F. Risk factors for rebleeding of aneurysmal subarachnoid hemorrhage: a meta-analysis. *PLoS One.* 2014;9(6):e99536.

[17] C. A. Hellingman, W. M. van den Bergh, I. S. Beijer, G. W. van Dijk, A. Algra, G. J. van, G. J. Rinkel. Risk of rebleeding after treatment of acute hydrocephalus in patients with aneurysmal subarachnoid hemorrhage. *Stroke*, 38 (2007), pp. 96–99.

[18] J. I. McIver, J. A. Friedman, E. F. Wijdicks, D. G. Piepgras, M. A. Pichelmann, L. G. Toussaint III, R. L. McClelland, D. A. Nichols, J. L. Atkinson. Preoperative ventriculostomy and rebleeding after aneurysmal subarachnoid hemorrhage. *J. Neurosurg.,* 97 (2002), pp. 1042–1044.

[19] L. Pare, R. Delfino, R. Leblanc. The relationship of ventricular drainage to aneurysmal rebleeding. *J. Neurosurg.,* 76 (1992), pp. 422–427.

[20] A. C. Ruijs, C. M. Dirven, A. Algra, I. Beijer, W. P. Vandertop, G. Rinkel. The risk of rebleeding after external lumbar drainage in patients with untreated ruptured cerebral aneurysms. *Acta Neurochir.* (Wien), 147 (2005), pp. 1157–1161.

[21] Beck, J., Rohde, S., el Beltagy, M., et al.: Difference in configuration of ruptured and unruptured intracranial aneurysms determined by biplanar digital subtraction angiography. *Acta Neurochir.* (Wien) 145:861–865, 2003.

[22] Hademenos, G. J., Massoud, T. F., Turjman, F., et al.: Anatomical and morphological factors correlating with rupture of intracranial aneurysms in patients referred for endovascular treatment. *Neuroradiology* 40:755–760, 1998

[23] Ma, B., Harbaugh, R. E., Raghavan, M. L: Three-dimensional geometrical characterization of cerebral aneurysms. *Ann. Biomed. Eng*. 32:264–273, 2004.

[24] A Stijntje E. Bor, Marieke, J. H. Wermer, Gabriel J. E. Rinkel. (2010) Unruptured intracranial aneurysms: initial and follow-up screening. *Future Neurology* 5:3, 421-431. Online publication date: 1-May-2010.

[25] Antovic, J., Bakic, M., Zivkovic, M., Ilic, A., Blomback, M. Blood coagulation and fibrinolysis in acute ischaemic and haemorrhagic (intracerebral and subarachnoid haemorrhage) stroke: does decreased plasmin inhibitor indicate increased fibrinolysis in subarachnoid haemorrhage compared to other types of stroke? *Scand. J. Clin. Lab. Invest.* 2002;62(3):195-9.

[26] Pliego, L. A., Muchnik, S. Fibrinolytic and factor XIII activity in subarachnoid hemorrhage. *Arq. Neuropsiquiatr.* 1997;55(3A):420-2.

[27] Roos, Y., Rinkel, G., Vermeulen, M., Algra, A., van Gijn, J. Antifibrinolytic therapy for aneurysmal subarachnoid hemorrhage: a major update of a cochrane review. *Stroke*. 2003;34(9):2308-9.

[28] Tsementzis, S. A., Honan, W. P., Nightingale, S., Hitchcock, E. R., Meyer CH. Fibrinolytic activity after subarachnoid haemorrhage and the effect of tranexamic acid. *Acta Neurochir.* (Wien). 1990;103(3-4):116-21.

[29] Juvela, S., Kaste, M. Reduced platelet aggregability and thromboxane release after rebleeding in patients with subarachnoid hemorrhage. *J. Neurosurg.* 1991;74(1):21-6.

[30] Ilveskero, S., Juvela, S., Siironen, J., Lassila, R. D-dimer predicts outcome after aneurysmal subarachnoid hemorrhage: no effect of thromboprophylaxis on coagulation activity. *Neurosurgery.* 2005;57(1):16-24; discussion 16-24.

[31] Morga, R., Czepko, R., Dembinska-Kiec, A., Danilewicz, B. Assessment of the haemostatic system in patients surgically treated for ruptured cerebral aneurysm. *Neurol. Neurochir. Pol.* 2007;41(4):296-305.

[32] Nina, P., Schisano, G., Chiappetta, F., Luisa, Papa M., Maddaloni, E., Brunori, A., et al. A study of blood coagulation and fibrinolytic system in spontaneous subarachnoid hemorrhage. Correlation with hunt-hess grade and outcome. *Surg. Neurol.* 2001;55(4):197-203.

[33] Peltonen, S., Juvela, S., Kaste, M., Lassila, R. Hemostasis and fibrinolysis activation after subarachnoid hemorrhage. *J. Neurosurg.* 1997;87(2):207-14.

[34] Chwajol, M., Starke, R. M., Kim, G. H., Mayer, S. A., Connolly, E. S. Antifibrinolytic therapy to prevent early rebleeding after subarachnoid hemorrhage. *Neurocrit. Care*. 2008;8(3):418-26.

[35] Starke, R. M., Kim, G. H., Fernandez, A., Komotar, R. J., Hickman, Z. L., Otten, M. L., et al. Impact of a protocol for acute antifibrinolytic therapy on aneurysm rebleeding after subarachnoid hemorrhage. *Stroke.* 2008;39(9):2617-21.

[36] Vermeij, F. H., Hasan, D., Bijvoet, H. W., Avezaat, C. J. Impact of medical treatment on the outcome of patients after aneurysmal subarachnoid hemorrhage. *Stroke*. 1998;29(5):924-30.

[37] Leipzig, T. J., Redelman, K., Horner, T. G. Reducing the risk of rebleeding before early aneurysm surgery: a possible role for antifibrinolytic therapy. *J. Neurosurg.* 1997;86(2):220-5.

[38] Post, R., Coert, B. A., Vandertop, W. P., Verbaan, D., Germans, M. R. Letter to the Editor: Short-term epsilon-aminocaproic acid treatment and endovascular coil embolization. *J. Neurosurg*. 2016:1-2.

[39] Kassell, N. F., Torner, J. C., Adams, H. P., Jr. Antifibrinolytic therapy in the acute period following aneurysmal subarachnoid hemorrhage. Preliminary observations from the Cooperative Aneurysm Study. *J. Neurosurg.* 1984;61(2):225-30.

[40] Harrigan, M. R., Rajneesh, K. F., Ardelt, A. A., Fisher, W. S., 3rd. Short-term antifibrinolytic therapy before early aneurysm treatment in subarachnoid hemorrhage: effects on rehemorrhage, cerebral ischemia, and hydrocephalus. *Neurosurgery.* 2010;67(4):935-9; discussion 9-40.

[41] Foreman, P. M., Chua, M., Harrigan, M. R., Fisher, W. S., 3rd, Tubbs, R. S., Shoja, M. M., et al. Antifibrinolytic therapy in aneurysmal subarachnoid hemorrhage increases the risk for deep venous thrombosis: A case-control study. *Clin. Neurol. Neurosurg.* 2015;139:66-9.

[42] Malekpour, M., Kulwin, C., Bohnstedt, B. N., Radmand, G., Sethia, R., Mendenhall, S. K., et al. Effect of short-term epsilon-aminocaproic acid treatment on patients undergoing endovascular coil embolization following aneurysmal subarachnoid hemorrhage. *J. Neurosurg.* 2016:1-8.

[43] Dunn, C. J., Goa, K. L. Tranexamic acid: a review of its use in surgery and other indications. *Drugs.* 1999;57(6):1005-32.

[44] Hardy, J. F., Belisle, S., Dupont, C., Harel, F., Robitaille, D., Roy, M., et al. Prophylactic tranexamic acid and epsilon-aminocaproic acid for primary myocardial revascularization. *Ann Thorac. Surg.* 1998;65(2):371-6.

[45] Fodstad, H., Kok, P., Algers, G. Fibrinolytic activity of cerebral tissue after experimental subarachnoid haemorrhage: inhibitory effect of tranexamic acid (AMCA). *Acta Neurol. Scand.* 1981;64(1):29-46.

[46] Germans, M. R., Post, R., Coert, B. A., Rinkel, G. J., Vandertop, W. P., Verbaan D. Ultra-early tranexamic acid after subarachnoid hemorrhage (ULTRA): study protocol for a randomized controlled trial. *Trials.* 2013;14:143.

[47] Baharoglu, M. I.1, Germans, M. R., Rinkel, G. J., Algra, A., Vermeulen, M., van Gijn, J., Roos Y. B. Antifibrinolytic therapy for aneurysmal subarachnoid haemorrhage. *Cochrane Database Syst. Rev.* 2013 Aug 30; (8): CD001245.

[48] Molyneux, A. J.1, Kerr, R. S., Yu, L. M., Clarke, M., Sneade, M., Yarnold, J. A., Sandercock, P.; International Subarachnoid Aneurysm Trial (ISAT) Collaborative Group. International subarachnoid aneurysm trial (ISAT) of neurosurgical clipping versus endovascular coiling in 2143 patients with ruptured intracranial aneurysms: a randomised comparison of effects on survival, dependency, seizures, rebleeding, subgroups, and aneurysm occlusion. *Lancet*. 2005 Sep 3-9; 366(9488):809-17.

INDEX

C

D

E

F

G

H

I

J

L

M

T

U

V

W

Y